STAY RIGHT WHERE YOU ARE

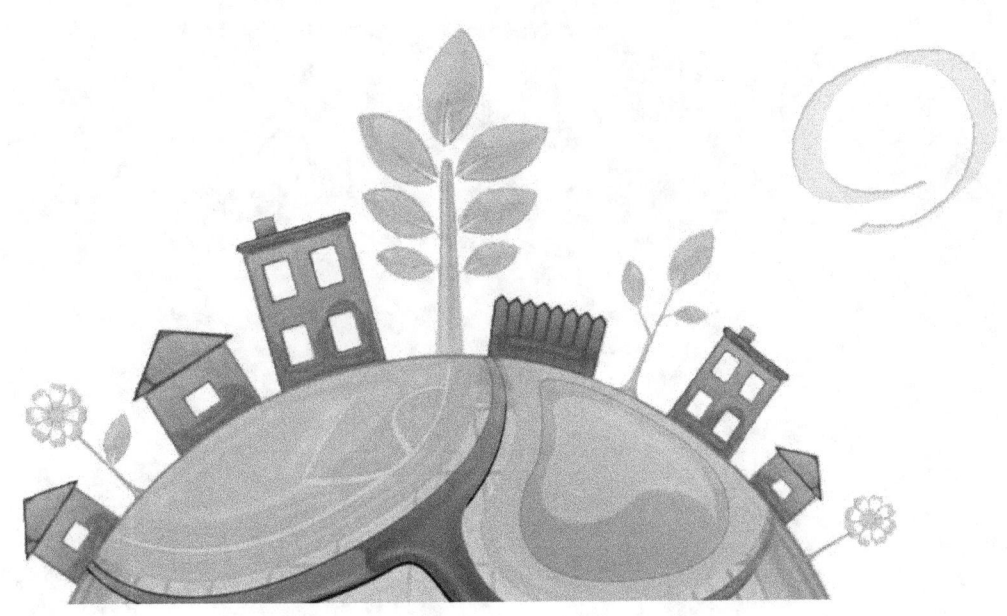

Resources for Seniors and
Adults with Disabilities Living at Home
in Washington State

Published by

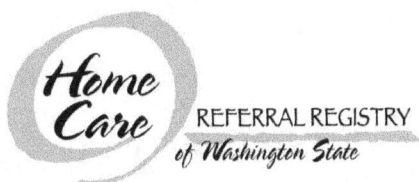

Stay Right Where You Are

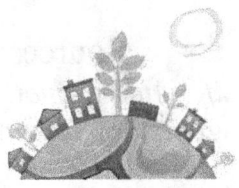

Resources for Seniors and
Adults with Disabilities Living at Home
in Washington State

Published by

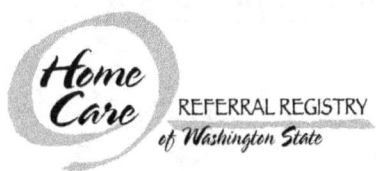

Home Care REFERRAL REGISTRY of Washington State

2009

Acknowledgements

Research and design by Grier Jewell

Thanks to the following individuals for their assistance with review:

- Debbie Johnson, Division of Developmental Disabilities, DSHS
- Dennis Mahar, LMTAAA Executive Director, DSHS
- Ann Vining, Attorney at law, Northwest Justice Project
- Jody McInturff, Aging and Disabilities Services Administration, DSHS
- Susan Shepherd, Aging and Disabilities Services Administration, DSHS

Sources:

Stay Active and Independent for Life: An Information Guide for Adults 65+, published by the Washington State Department of Health

Medicaid and Long Term Care Services for Adults, published by the Washington State Department of Social and Health Services

Table of Contents

INTRODUCTION

Stay Right Where You Are is a basic guide for seniors and adults with disabilities who want to continue living at home and need help to make that happen.

The amount of information on services and supports for seniors and adults with disabilities can be a lot to sort through.

If you're dealing with complex medical issues, government agencies or insurance companies, getting help can be downright overwhelming.

Think of this guide as a map made up of helpful people.

They might be part of a small community program or a government agency with a ten-dollar title, but they all share one thing in common:

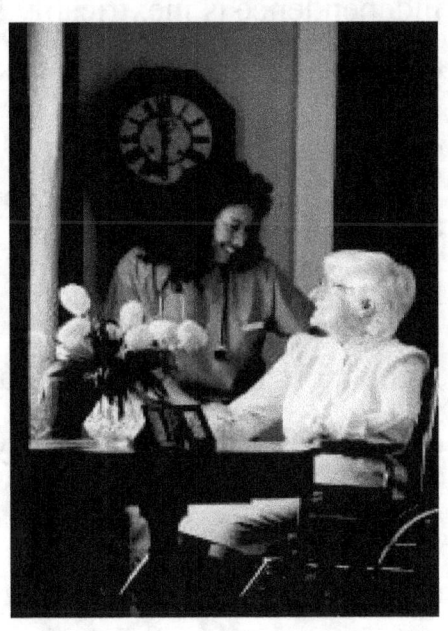

They want to help you live in your own home.

Regardless of age or disability, there are services and supports to help you stay as independent as possible.

So, stay right where you are. Skip, flip, or read through this guide to find people with the help you need to keep living in your own home.

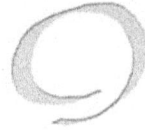

Lay of the Land

At some point in life, we all face transitions that cause us to look outside ourselves for help. Whether it's due to age or disability, the ability to maintain our independence is inextricably linked to receiving support and services—from a little to a lot.

The good news is that there's an abundance of options to help adults of all ages and abilities remain at home. The downside is that so many services can make it hard to find the right one(s).

If the thought of sorting through the vast universe of service systems and community programs makes your head spin, you're not alone. *Making life easier is hard work for everyone.*

This guide can't simplify the world of home and community support, but it can start you on your journey with some basic resources and people to help you figure out what you need.

Each of the five sections are designed to point you toward:

✿ **Getting Started**

✿ **Help at Home**

✿ **Help in the Community**

✿ **Taking Care of Business**

✿ **Directory of Resources**

GETTING STARTED

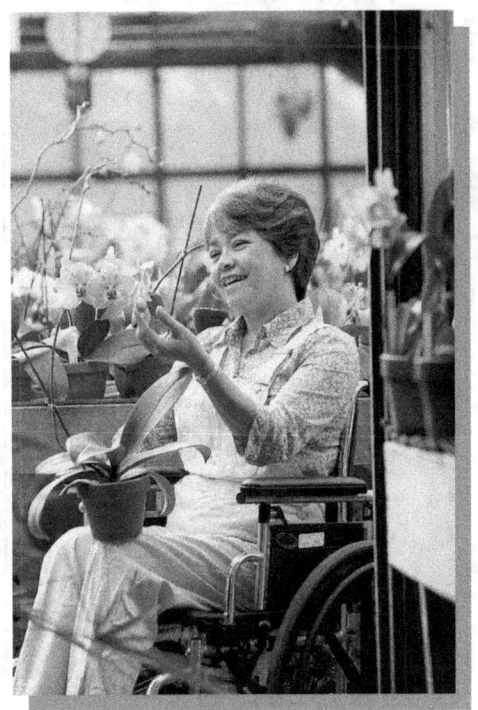

Assess Your Needs and Resources: Identify the kinds of things that will help you be as independent as possible.

Benefits Check-Up: The fastest, easiest way to match your needs and resources with available services.

Where to Go…Who to Call: Key contacts for people age 60 and older and adults with disabilities under age 60.

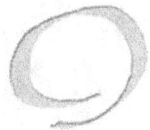

Assess Your Needs and Resources

Make a list of the things you need help with, or things you can't do as well as you once could.

Don't leave anything off your list.

Letting some things go—like housecleaning and cooked meals—can put your health and safety at risk and hinder your independence.

Next, gather your financial information. This includes:

- All sources of your income (such as Social Security, pensions, employment, cash assistance programs);

- Expenses (including out-of-pocket costs for medical expenses not covered by health insurance, rent or mortgage, heating fuel, gas, electricity, water, telephone;

- Assets (cash, bank accounts, stocks, bonds, CDs, second car);

Things I Need

✓ A ride to the doctor

✓ Lawn care

✓ Help getting dressed

✓ Prescription drug coverage

✓ Help with the electric bill

✓ Someone to check in on me

✓ Meals delivered

✓ Wheelchair ramp

- The financial information of anyone else in your family who shares financial responsibility.

If you'd like to have someone help you in person, the next few pages will get you pointed in the right direction.

GETTING STARTED

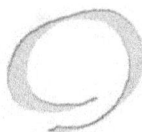

Benefits Check Up

Benefit's Check Up (a service of the National Council on Aging) is the nation's most comprehensive Web-based service used to screen for benefits programs.

It provides information on more than 1,550 public and private benefits programs, such as:

✿ Prescription drugs

✿ Nutrition

✿ Energy assistance

✿ Financial aide

✿ Legal assistance

✿ Health care

✿ Social Security benefits

✿ Housing

✿ In-home services

✿ Tax relief

✿ Transportation

✿ Educational assistance

HOW IT WORKS

BenefitsCheckUp.org provides a list of services for which you may qualify based on your income, resources, medical or physical needs.

After you answer all the questions, you will be provided a list of people to contact for help.

It's easy to do and takes about 20-30 minutes to complete.

Benefits Check Up

Find out what kind of benefits you may qualify for, based on your needs and income:

www.benefitscheckup.org

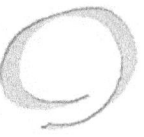

Where to Go... Who to Call

For People Age 60 and Older

Senior Information and Assistance (typically known as I & A) is a free information and referral service for adults 60 and over and for family and friends helping care for the older adult.

I&A services are provided through your local Area Agency on Aging (AAA).

Contact your AAA any time you have a question about getting help for an adult sixty or older.

Senior I&A Helps You

○ plan, find and get more care, services, or programs (e.g. transportation, meals, housekeeping, personal care);

○ explore options for paying for long term care and review eligibility for benefits;

○ figure out health care insurance and prescription drug options;

○ sort through legal issues (such as setting up advance directives, living wills)

HOW TO FIND YOUR LOCAL AREA AGENCY ON AGING (AAA)

For the AAA office nearest you, see page 105-107 in the Government Directory of this guide.

Or, visit the Department of Social and Health Services (DSHS) Aging and Disabilities Services Administration (ADSA) website:

www.adsa.dshs.wa.gov

(Click on Find Local Services for a statewide map.)

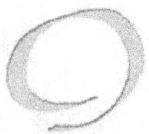

Where to Go...
Who to Call

For People with Disabilities Under Age 60

Home and Community Services (HCS) is the best place to start if you're under age 60 and need help living in your home due to a disability.

HCS is a division of the Department of Social and Health Services (DSHS) Aging and Disability Services Administration (ADSA).

HCS will determine if you're eligible to receive services such as Medicaid Personal Care (MPC) or additional community-based services.

If you're eligible for home and community-based services, case management will be provided through your local Area Agency on Aging (AAA). But your first stop is at HCS.

[Note: If you have a developmental disability, you can also contact your local Division of Developmental Disabilities. See the following page for more information.]

To find out if you're eligible for in-home services, contact the Home and Community Services office nearest you.

For a listing of local numbers, see page 110 in the Government Directory of this guide.

Or, visit the Department of Social and Health Services (DSHS) Aging and Disabilities Services Administration (ADSA) website:

www.adsa.dshs.wa.gov

(Click on Find Local Services for a statewide map.)

GETTING STARTED

GETTING STARTED

Independent Living Centers

are non-profit, non-residential centers run by persons with disabilities.

Depending on the area, some of the services they offer may include:

✿ Information and
   Referral

✿ Peer Support

✿ Independent Living Skills Training

✿ Individual Advocacy

✿ Systems Advocacy

✿ Benefits Counseling

✿ Housing Referrals

✿ Legal Aid

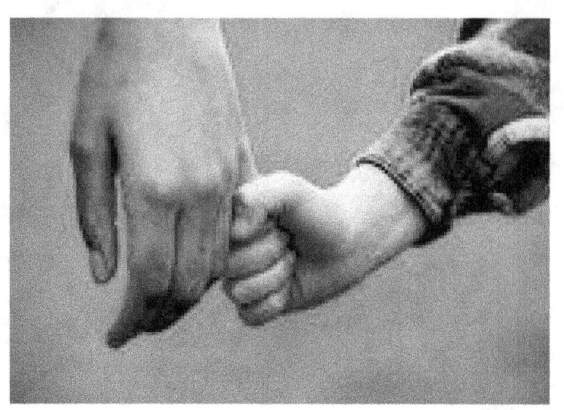

Services for People with Developmental Disabilities

Adults with developmental disabilities have the option of going to the Division of Developmental Disabilities (DDD) where they may be eligible to receive services such as employment, Medicaid Personal Care (MPC), supported living, therapies, and respite.

For a list of regional DDD offices, see page 109 in the Government Directory of this guide. Or, call the Aging and Disabilities Services Administration Helpline:

☎   **1-800-422-3263**

☎   **1-800-737-7931 (TDD)**

For a list of Independent Living Centers throughout the state, see page 92 in the Topical Directory of this guide under *Disability*.

Or, visit the Washington State Independent Living Council website:

💻   **www.wasilc.org**

(Click on the link for Independent Living Centers in the left column.)

HELP AT HOME

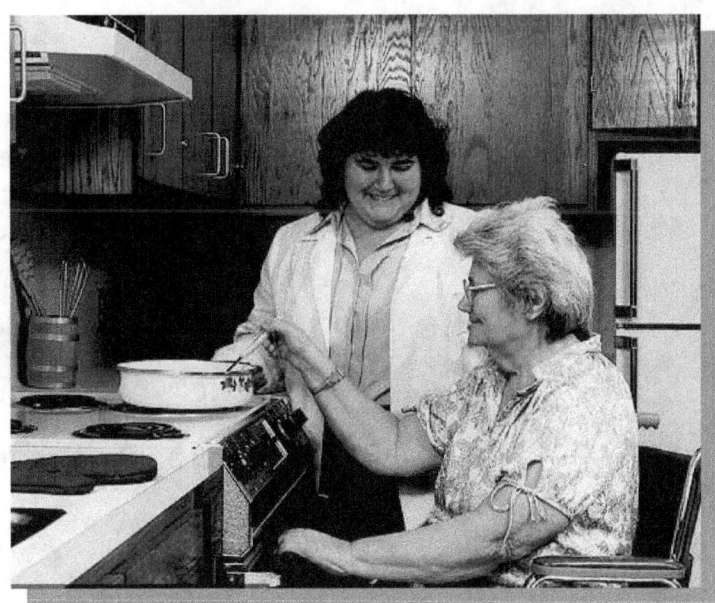

In-Home Care: How to find services to help you live as independently as possible.

Help for Helpers: Support groups, respite and resources for unpaid helpers.

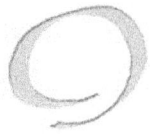

In-Home Care

If you need help taking care of personal needs such as bathing, dressing, and preparing meals—or have a health condition that requires professional medical assistance—you don't have to move out of your home to get the services you need.

Whether you pay out of your own pocket for a few hours of personal care or qualify for services through Medicaid, Medicare, or private insurance, you can stay right where you are. Help will come to you.

The following pages describe the different options for receiving in-home services:

✿ Personal Care

✿ Community Options Program Entry System (COPES)

✿ Volunteer Chore Services

✿ Services for Persons with Developmental Disabilities

✿ Medicaid Nurse Delegation

✿ Home Health/Skilled Nursing

✿ Hospice

Home Care and Home Health

What's the Difference?

It's easy to confuse Home Care services with Home Health services. When applying for services, here's a simple way to understand the type of services you may be eligible to receive:

Home Care is a non-medical in-home service such as help with bathing, dressing, eating, or toileting. Personal care is an example of Home Care.

Home Health includes medically necessary services such as skilled nursing; physical therapy; home infusion therapy; wound care; or health aide services.

Personal Care

In-home personal care is for people who need help with things like taking a bath, toileting, getting dressed, preparing meals, eating, and transferring in and out of a wheelchair (to name just a few things considered "personal care").

Individual care providers can be hired as part-time, full-time, or live-in caregivers. They can also be hired as back-up to your regular caregiver.

You can pay for personal care out of your own pocket or through public funding if you meet income eligibility.

Who Provides Personal Care?

Individuals who provide in-home personal care can be hired directly (as independent care providers) or through an agency.

Independent Care Providers

State contracted in-home caregivers are called Individual Providers (IPs). IPs are employed as caregivers by people who use Medicaid to help pay for needed care in their home.

Anyone can become paid personal care providers, including friends and family (with the exception of spouses), as well as parents of individuals with developmental disabilities 18 years and older.

For more information about finding an Individual Provider, contact the Home Care Referral Registry:

☎   **1-800-970-5456**

Agency Workers

Hundreds of home care agencies throughout the state recruit, hire, train and supervise in-home workers to provide personal care and respite services.

Whether you pay out of your own pocket or receive publicly funded services, you can choose to hire a home care worker through an agency. When you hire through an agency, the agency dispatches your care provider.

HELP AT HOME

Cost of Personal Care

Private Pay: If you're paying for personal care services yourself, expect to pay about $20-$22 per hour (average cost in 2008) for someone from a home care agency. Typically, there is a three or four hour per day minimum for services.

You can always pay someone who's not part of an agency to help you out at home, and you can negotiate the price of those services yourself.

Public Funding: Seniors and adults with disabilities who have been assessed to need help with activities of daily living (such as eating, bathing, toileting, transfers, and getting dressed) may qualify for Medicaid Personal Care services at little or no cost (depending on your income).

How to Apply for Personal Care: Contact Home and Community Services (HCS) and request an application.

For the number of the HCS office nearest you, see page 110 in the Government Directory of this guide. Or, apply for Medicaid online through the Department of Social and Health Services (DSHS) Aging and Disabilities Services Administration (ADSA) website:

💻   **www.adsa.dshs.wa.gov**

(Click on "Apply for Medicaid.)

If you have a developmental disability, you can also apply for Medicaid Personal Care (MPC) and other services through the Division of Developmental Disabilities (DDD). For the number of the DDD office nearest you, see page 109 in the Government Directory of this guide, or call the Aging and Disability Services Administration Helpline:

☎   **1-800-422-3263**

For more information on paying for services, see **Taking Care of Business—Paying for Services** on page 51 of this guide.

How to Find Individual Providers:

If you are eligible to receive Medicaid in-home care services, the Home Care Referral Registry can help you explore ways to find and hire an Individual Provider (IP) who's most suited to your needs.

The Home Care Referral Registry can match your in-home care needs with pre-qualified, pre-screened individual providers that are ready to work. For a list of prescreened IPs call:

☎ **1-800-970-5456**

How to Find Home Care Agencies

Look in the Yellow Pages of the phone book, under Home Health Care and Services.

Or, visit the following websites:

National Association of Home Care Agencies: www.nahc.org (Click on Consumer Info)

The Home Care Association of Washington: www.hcaw.org

How to Hire a Care Provider

Once you have a list of names you will need to call and see who might be right for an interview.

Before You Interview:

✿ Identify number of days/week and hours/day needed.

✿ Identify the job duties (ex. Meal preparation, dressing, bathing, transportation, etc.)

Interview Questions:

✿ Do you have previous experience as a caregiver?

✿ Where have you worked before? How long were you there and why did you leave?

✿ Can you perform the duties required for this position?

✿ Is there anything I described that you are uncomfortable with?

✿ Do you have a driver's license and reliable transportation?

✿ Can you perform the duties required for this position?

✿ Can you give me two references?

HELP AT HOME

HELP AT HOME

Community Options Program Entry System (COPES)

If you need more than personal care to help you live in your home, and you are eligible for Medicaid, additional services can be provided through the Community Options Program Entry System (COPES).

In addition to Personal Care, COPES pays for:

o   Home Modification;

o   Personal Emergency Response System;

o   Adult Day Care/Day Health;

o   Transportation;

o   Home Delivered Meals;

o   Medical Equipment;

o   Skilled Nursing.

Eligibility for COPES is based on income and assessed need for help with activities of daily living.

To be eligible for COPES in 2009, your income must be no more than $2,022 per month if you are single. If you're married, and your income is not more than $2,022, you may be eligible no matter how much income your spouse makes. (Income limits change annually.)

If you're married and your income is more than $2,022, you may still be eligible for COPES if the sum of your income and your spouse's income is less than $4,044. [Source: Columbia Legal Services, Questions and Answers on the COPES Program, 2009.]

To download Questions and Answers on COPES: visit the Washington Law Help website:

🖥   **www.washingtonlawhelp.org**

(Click on the icon for Government Benefits, then click on Long Term Care Assistance)

A separate program covers in-home care for some individuals whose income is above $2,022 (for 2009). It's called the Medically Needy In-home Waiver or MNIW.

As with all of these services, contact the appropriate agency for more information.

[See page 66 for legal resources if you've been denied services and would like to appeal that decision.]

Cost: If your income exceeds Federal Poverty Level (FPL), you will be required to pay for some of the cost of COPES services.

[For 2009, the FPL is $10,830 for a single person household.]

The amount you pay will depend on your income. People receiving Supplemental Security Income (SSI) do not pay.

How to Apply: Contact Home and Community Services (HCS). For the number of the HCS office nearest you, see page 110 in the Government Directory of this guide, or visit:

💻   **www.adsa.dshs.wa.gov**

(Click on Find Local Services)

Volunteer Chore Services

Volunteer chore services are for adults with low-income who can't afford to pay for in-home services but don't qualify for other state assistance.

Volunteers can help with things like household chores, shopping, moving, minor home repair, yard care, personal care, and transportation.

Cost: Free to low-income adults who don't qualify for other state assistance.

How to Apply: Contact AAA. For a list of your local AAA see page 105-107 in the Government Directory of this guide, or visit:

💻   **www.adsa.dshs.wa.gov**

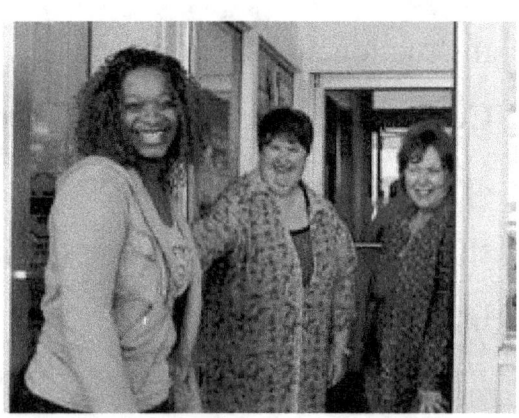

HELP AT HOME

HELP AT HOME

Services for Adults with Developmental Disabilities

Adults with developmental disabilities who require more support and supervision than Medicaid Personal Care provides, may be able to receive non-facility based services through the following programs:

Companion Homes

Companion Homes provide residential services and supports in an adult foster care model to no more than one adult who's a client of the Division of Developmental Disabilities (DDD).

The services are offered in a regular family residence approved by DDD to assure client health, safety, and well-being.

DDD reimburses the provider for the instruction and support service. Companion homes provide 24-hour available supervision. Services are subject to available funding (waiting list may apply).

Supported Living

Supported living services help people with developmental disabilities learn how to do things for themselves, such as cooking, cleaning, shopping, personal hygiene and paying bills.

Services are provided through a Medicaid Home and Community Based waiver program for eligible clients of DDD and are subject to being placed on a waiver (waivers are currently at capacity, Fall 2008).

Supported living services are provided in the individual's own home or apartment (typically shared with one to three other people).

Supports may vary from a few hours per month up to 24 hours per day of one-to-one (or shared) support. The Division of Developmental Disabilities (DDD) contracts with private agencies to provide Supported Living services.

Cost: Services are covered by Medicaid; however, rent, food, utilities and personal expenses are paid by the individual (typically, this is paid for with the individual's Supplemental Security Income payments).

To Apply: Contact the Division of Developmental Disabilities.

See page 109 in the Government Directory of this guide, for a listing of regional DDD offices.

Medicaid Nurse Delegation

In the past, many people had to move to a nursing home if health care services were needed from a licensed health care professional such as a registered nurse (RN).

With the Nurse Delegation Program, it's possible to get help with certain health care tasks from an unlicensed caregiver at home.

If you receive Medicaid and have nursing care needs, your Case Manager will make a referral to a registered nurse (RN) who has contracted with DSHS to perform nurse delegation services.

Once the referral is made, you meet with an RN for an evaluation of your health care needs. Your condition must be "stable and predictable" and the RN must feel confident that your caregiver will be able to do the task(s) safely.

The RN will work directly with your caregiver(s) and train him or her to do the task(s) safely and correctly.

Your caregiver must be registered with the state as a nursing assistant, receive training, and be approved by the RN before assisting with any health care tasks. Through Nurse Delegation, your caregiver can:

o Give you prescription medications as ordered;

o Test your blood sugar levels (if you have a long standing medical condition such as diabetes);

o Perform tube feedings, bladder emptying, special bowel programs, and simple wound care.

NOTE: With the exception of insulin injections, a nurse cannot delegate injections, perform procedures that are considered sterile, or tasks that require nursing judgment.

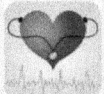 **Making Healthy Choices**

Improve Your Mental Fitness

✿ Keep up your social life.

✿ Read a variety of newspapers, magazines and books.

✿ Play games like Scrabble, cards, cross word puzzles and Chess.

✿ Take a class on a subject that interests you.

✿ Begin a new hobby.

✿ Learn a new language.

How to apply for Nurse Delegation:

Talk with your case manager if you are interested in learning more about the Nurse Delegation Program and are currently receiving Medicaid.

Home Health/Skilled Nursing

If you have complex health care needs that cannot be delegated by a nurse, or if you recently suffered an injury or illness that required hospitalization or care in a nursing home, you may be able to receive home health services through:

o Medicaid COPES or Medically Needy In-Home Waiver

o Private insurance and Medicare (under limited conditions)

o Private Pay

Individuals requiring skilled home health services usually receive their care from a home health agency.

Some agencies deliver a variety of in-home services through nurses, therapists, social workers, aides, durable medical equipment dealers, and volunteers.

Many home health agencies are Medicare-certified and contracted to receive Medicare and Medicaid reimbursement.

Home Health Services Include:

Skilled Nursing; Physical Therapy; Speech Therapy; Home Infusion Therapy; Wound Care; or Health Aide Services.

How to Apply for Home Health through Medicaid:

Contact Home and Community Services (HCS). To find the number of the HCS office nearest you, see page 110 in the Government Directory of this guide or call the Aging and Disability Services Administration Helpline:

   1-800-422-3263

Hospice Care

Hospice care provides comprehensive medical, psychological, and spiritual care for people who are terminally ill, as well as support for patients' families. It's based primarily in the home, enabling families to remain together.

Trained hospice professionals are available 24-hours a day to assist the

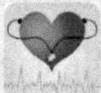 **Making Healthy Choices**

Recognize the Signs of Depression

✿ An "empty" feeling, ongoing sadness, and anxiety

✿ Tiredness, lack of energy

✿ Sleep problems, including trouble getting to sleep, very early morning waking, and sleeping too much

✿ Eating more or less than usual

✿ Crying too often or too much

✿ Aches and pains that don't go away when treated

✿ A hard time focusing, remembering, or making decisions

✿ Feeling guilty, helpless, worthless, or hopeless

✿ Thoughts of death or suicide, a suicide attempt

family in caring for the patient, ensure that the patient's wishes are honored, and keep the patient comfortable and free from pain. Most hospices are Medicare-certified and licensed according to state requirements.

Cost: Hospice services are covered

HELP AT HOME

under the Medicare Hospice Benefit, Medicaid Hospice Benefit, and by most private insurers.

Additional Resources

The Washington State Hospice & Palliative Care Organization provides an online statewide search tool for hospice agencies and palliative care programs:

☎　　1-866-661-3739

-OR-

🖥　　www.wshpco.org

The Home Care Association of Washington online directory can help you find and choose an agency that provides home care and hospice services.

The database consists of home care and hospice agencies that are members of the Home Care Association of Washington.

🖥　　www.hcaw.org

HOME CARE REFERRAL REGISTRY

If you are eligible to receive Medicaid in-home care services, the Home Care Referral Registry can help you explore ways to find and hire an Individual Provider (IP) who's most suited to your needs.

The Home Care Referral Registry can match your in-home care needs with pre-qualified, pre-screened individual providers that are ready to work.

Once you've hired an IP, you'll need to contact your case worker at HCS, AAA, or DDD to ensure your IP has a DSHS contract before the IP begins working with you.

For more information, contact the Home Care Referral Registry:

☎　　1-800-970-5456

🖥　　www.hcrr.wa.gov

Home Care REFERRAL REGISTRY *of Washington State*

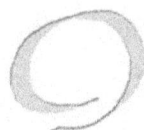

Help for Helpers

If you're helping a friend or family member get the support he or she needs, it's important to find support for yourself as well.

Respite Care

Respite care is a service where another trained person provides planned, short-term care (a few hours to a few days) in order to give you a break from caregiving.

Respite care can be arranged through adult day health or adult day care programs, family, friends, and volunteers.

Private pay—If you're paying for respite services out of your own pocket, and would like to hire someone from an agency, expect to pay about $20-$22 per hour (2008 average cost).

However, if you choose to hire an individual who's not part of an

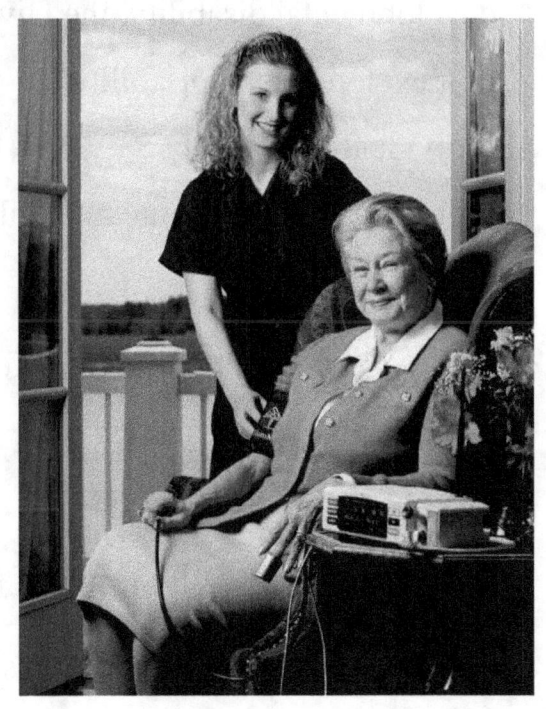

agency, you can negotiate payment.

You can also pay for Adult Day services, which provide respite at an hourly rate that ranges from $10-12 per hour (2008 average costs).

[Note: Depending on the organization that offers the services, there may be a three or four hour daily minimum.]

Publicly-funded—Volunteer Chore provides respite to non-paid caregivers of individuals with low-income on a limited basis.

For non-paid family caregivers who live with a family member who has a developmental disability, the Division of Developmental Disability's Individual and Family Services (IFS) program provides respite to eligible family caregivers.

Senior Companion programs offer respite to anyone regardless of income.

Caregiver Training

Powerful Tools for Caregiving is an educational series developed specifically for family members caring for someone with a chronic illness.

Powerful Tools for Caregiving shares a variety of self-care tools and strategies to reduce your stress, deal with difficult feelings, and make tough caregiving decisions.

To find out if *Powerful Tools for Caregiving* is available in your area, contact your local Area Agency on

Aging.

You can find a list of local AAA's on page 105-107 in the Government Directory of this guide, or by visiting the Aging and Disabilities Services Administration (ADSA) website:

www.adsa.dshs.wa.gov

(Click on Find Local Services for a statewide map.)

Free Resource Book:

Family Caregiver Handbook is published by the Washington State Department of Social and Health Services.

It includes information on:

✿ The Emotional Challenges of Caregiving

✿ Where to Turn When You Need Help

To order a copy, email:

fulfillment@prt.wa.gov

Or call **360-570-3062**.

Be sure to include the following publication number in your request: DSHS 22-277(x).

DSHS Required Training for Paid Providers

Are you looking for information about required DSHS training?

To register for the Revised Fundamentals of Caregiving, contact your local Area Agency on Aging (see page 105-107 in the Government Directory of this guide).

For all other training, contact the Aging and Disability Services Administration for more information:

ADSA Helpline:

1-800-422-3263

ADSA Website:
www.adsa.dshs.wa.gov

(Click on the left hand link to Professionals and Providers)

- **Nurse Delegation**
- **Revised Fundamentals of Caregiving**
- **Specialty Training in Developmental Disabilities, Mental Health and Dementia**
- **Parent Provider Training (6 -hour training for parents of adults with developmental disabilities)**

HELP AT HOME

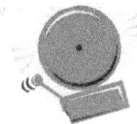

Signs that You May Need Help

From the *Caregiver Handbook*, published by
the Washington State Aging and Disability Services Administration

There are some occasions where the stress of caregiving puts you at risk of harming yourself or your loved one.

If you experience any of these symptoms on the right, you are carrying too great a burden.

Consider professional counseling or talk to your doctor about your feelings.

Your doctor may recommend a counselor, or you can contact your local hospital, Mental Health Department, or the Yellow Pages to find a psychologist, social worker, counselor, or other mental health professional.

Danger signals may be:

✿ Using excessive amounts of alcohol or medications like sleeping pills.

✿ Loss of appetite or eating too much.

✿ Depression, loss of hope, feelings of alienation.

✿ Thoughts of suicide.

✿ Losing control physically or emotionally.

✿ Neglecting or treating the other person roughly.

Although it's hard to ask for help, it's even harder to provide care alone! It's not a sign of weakness to ask for help. Instead, it's an important step in making sure the care receiver gets the help he needs.

HELP AT HOME

Caring for Someone with Alzheimer's Disease (AD)

From the *Caregiver's Guide*, published by the National Institute on Aging
Alzheimer's Disease Education and Referral Center

Trying to communicate with a person who has Alzheimer's Disease (AD) can be a challenge. Both understanding and being understood may be difficult.

✿ Choose simple words and short sentences and use a gentle, calm tone of voice.

✿ Avoid talking to the person with AD like a baby or talking about the person as if he or she weren't there.

✿ Minimize distractions and noise—such as the television or radio—to help the person focus on what you are saying.

✿ Call the person by name, making sure you have his or her attention before speaking.

✿ Allow enough time for a response. Be careful not to interrupt.

✿ If the person with AD is struggling to find a word or communicate a thought, gently try to provide the word he or she is looking for.

✿ Try to frame questions and instructions in a positive way.

Additional Resources

Alzheimer's Association

Provides information, education and support. 24-Hour Helpline:

☎   **1.800.272.3900**

💻   **www.alz.org**

Alzheimer's Disease Education and Referral Center

The ADEAR Center is operated as a service of the National Institute on Aging (NIA). The NIA conducts and supports research about health issues for older people, and is the primary Federal agency for Alzheimer's disease research.

☎   **1-800-438-4380**

💻   **www.alzheimers.org**

Children of Aging Parents

A nonprofit membership organization that provides information and referral services for a variety of professionals, information about support groups, and educational outreach services.

💻   **www.caps4caregivers.org**

Caring From a Distance

Caring From a Distance is a nonprofit organization created by men and women dealing with long distance care.

💻   **www.cfad.org**

Family Care Navigator

State-by-State Help for Family Caregivers.

💻   **www.caregiver.org**

Empowering Caregivers

Empowering Caregivers offers a link to assistance, education, support and referrals for family members. Caregivers can subscribe to an email newsletter

as well as participate in chat
rooms and on-line message
boards.

💻   **www.care-givers.com**

Lotsa Helping Hands

As part of the National Family
Caregivers Association, Lotsa
Helping Hands is a free online
service for creating a private and
secure online web community to
organize informal support for
your loved one.

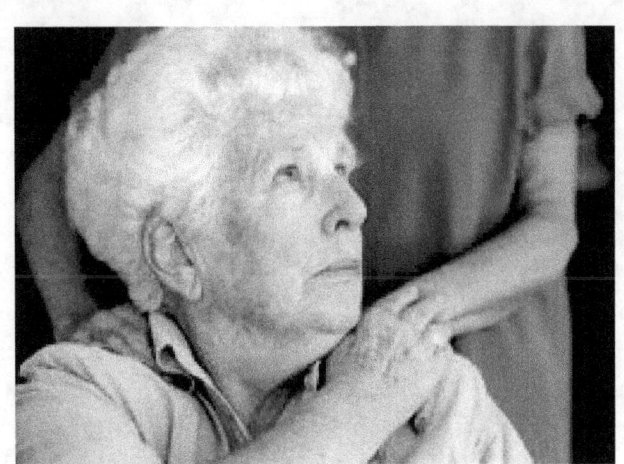

With no training, volunteers can
easily view and sign up for any
number of available tasks, review
their current commitments, and
be confident they won't forget
any assignments because the
system automatically sends out
email reminders of upcoming
obligations.

💻   **www.nfca.lotsahelping**

hands.com

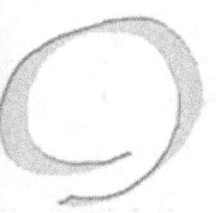

HELP IN THE COMMUNITY

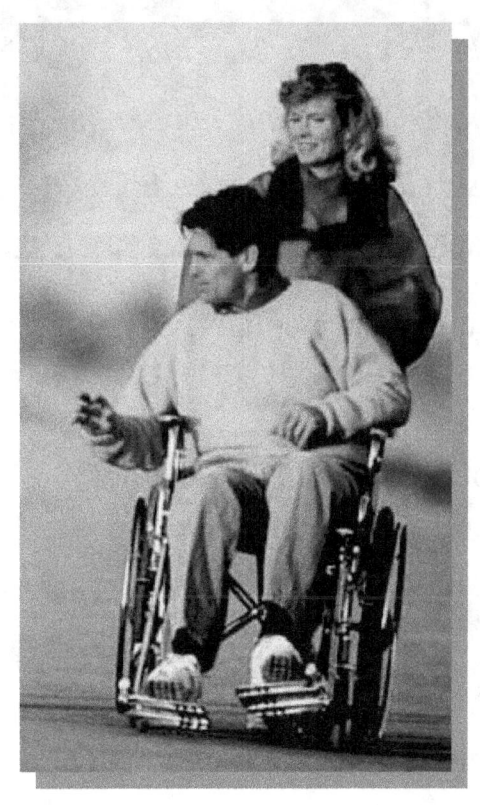

Community Programs: Learn about organizations in your community that offer free and low-cost programs to help you stay engaged and connected with others.

Community Health Programs: From prescription drugs to dental care, find health services that help fill in the gaps of medical coverage.

Transportation Options: Learn different options for getting around town.

Housing and Utilities: Learn about affordable housing and assistance with utility bills.

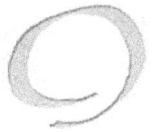 # Community Programs

If you're helping someone who's uncomfortable with the idea of accepting services and supports, start by looking close to home with informal support.

Senior centers, churches, temples, and charitable organizations offer a goldmine of resources and people who can help you figure out what's available in your local community.

Every area of the state is unique. The type of services offered to seniors and people with disabilities reflect the diverse needs and nature of each county, city and neighborhood.

The next few pages list the programs typically found in most communities throughout Washington.

> *"In talking to my parents about the services they needed, I might as well have been talking about going to the moon.*
>
> *So I started with people and places they were already familiar with, like their church, which has all kinds of help. That made it easier for them to think about other services later on."*   Anita G.

Adult Day Services

Adult day care is a daytime program for adults who need some level of care but not the same level of care provided by an RN or rehabilitative therapist. Services in most adult day care programs include help with personal care, social activities, classes, routine health monitoring, meals and snacks, coordination of transportation, first aid, and emergency care.

Adult day health is a daytime program for adults who need skilled

HELP IN THE COMMUNITY

nursing care or a licensed rehabilitative therapist. An adult day health center provides skilled nursing services, counseling, therapy (physical, occupational, speech, or audiology), personal care services, social services, general therapeutic activities, health education, nutritional meals and snacks, and supervision.

How to Pay: The typical cost for private pay ranges from $40-$65 per day, or an hourly rate of $10-$12 (2008 average estimated cost). Fees may be waived or reduced through

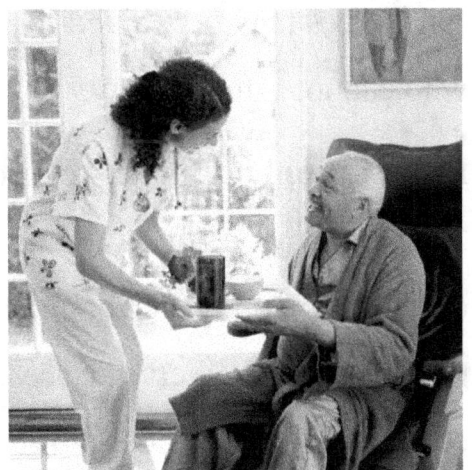

scholarships offered by some adult day service providers.

Adult Day Services may also be publicly-funded through programs such as Medicaid for individuals with low-income.

Note: Medicare does not pay for Adult Day Services.

To find the nearest Adult Day Services program, contact the **Washington Adult Day Services Association:**

    1-888-609-2372

Companion Programs

Senior Companions serve adults who need extra assistance to live independently in their own homes or communities.

These programs benefit older adults, adults with disabilities, those with terminal illnesses, and offer respite for caregivers.

There are four Senior Companion Programs in Washington State.

HELP IN THE COMMUNITY

Each program is sponsored by a local organization. Services vary depending on the needs of each area, but may include: help paying bills, help reading and writing, someone to visit and (in some areas) transportation.

How to Pay: Services are free to anyone.

Grays Harbor/Thurston and Pacific Counties:

☎   360-532-9542 or

☎   888-532-9542

King County:

☎   206-329-0515

Pierce/Kitsap Counties:

☎   253-272-8433

Yakima/Benton/Franklin Counties:

☎   509-946-4645

Meals and Food Assistance

Home Delivered Meals

Meal and nutrition programs are offered to seniors and persons with disabilities who are unable to leave their homes.

Programs vary greatly. Meal delivery programs, such as Meals on Wheels, are contracted with local agencies (such as a senior center).

How to Pay: For most meal delivery programs, eligible persons may be able to make voluntary donations toward the cost of the meals.

Basic Food Benefits, in the form of a Quest Card (see next page), may be accepted from participants as contributions toward the cost; and some individuals on COPES are authorized to receive home-delivered meals.

Cost is based on a sliding fee scale. Depending on the availability of funds, fees may be waived for people who cannot afford to pay.

How to Apply: Contact your local Area Agency on Aging to find the organization or agency contracted to provide meal delivery services. The contracting agency does a brief assessment to determine eligibility.

For a list of AAAs, see page 105-107

in the Government Directory of this guide, or visit:

⌨   **www.adsa.dshs.wa.gov**

(Click on Find Local Services)

Group Meals

Also known as congregate meals, group meals are offered at various community locations, such as a senior center, tribal center or community center.

How to Pay: Meals for persons age 60 and older are typically available through voluntary donations toward the cost of the meals. Basic Food Benefits might be accepted as contributions; and with some exceptions, persons under 60 would pay full price.

How to Apply: Just show up. You can get a list of on-site meal programs from your local Area Agency on Aging.

Washington Basic Food Program

Once known as "food stamps" this program issues Electronic Benefits Transfer (EBT) Cards, also called "Quest Cards." The Quest card is used like a debit card to purchase food items at stores.

How to Apply: Contact your local Community Services Office. For the number of the office nearest you, call the Aging and Disability Services Administration Helpline:

☎   **1-800-422-3263**

Or apply online:

⌨   **https://fortress.wa.gov/dshs/f2ws03esaapps/onlineapp/introduction_1.asp**

Food Banks

Hundreds of food banks exist throughout the state. No one is turned away.

How to Apply: Just show up.

To find a food bank near you, contact Northwest Harvest:

☎   **1-800-722-6924**

For a statewide map of food banks:

⌨   **www.cted.wa.gov/maps/**

HELP IN THE COMMUNITY

HELP IN THE COMMUNITY

Senior Farmers Market Nutrition Program

The Senior Farmers Market Nutrition provides fresh fruit and vegetables to seniors with lower income. It also supports local farming by increasing the use of farmers markets, roadside stands, and community supported agriculture.

Produce is also purchased directly from farmers for delivery to seniors. The program is funded by the U.S. Department of Agriculture (USDA), State of Washington funds, and some local area funds.

The program operates June through October.

Eligibility: Seniors whose income is below 185% of Federal Poverty Level, ($1,670/mo for one in 2009) AND who are age 60 and older.

How it works: Eligible seniors may use the program in one of two ways:

1. Redeem farmers market checks worth a total of $40 for produce at authorized farmers markets or roadside stands.

-OR-

2. Local produce is purchased directly from farmers and delivered to eligible homebound seniors or to meal sites and senior housing for pick up by seniors.

For information on how to apply for benefits, contact the program coordinator in your area (listed under "Meals & Food Assistance" in the Topical Directory of this guide).

Personal Emergency Response Systems

Home medical alert systems, sometimes called Personal Emergency Response Systems are very helpful for adults at risk for falling or who have a fear of falling; limited mobility; medication concerns; or medical conditions.

How it works:

An electronic device is provided that allows you to get help in an emergency.

The system is connected to your phone, or you can wear a portable "help" button.

When activated, staff at a response center will call 911 or take whatever action has been pre-arranged by the subscriber (such as calling people you've identified as emergency contacts).

Cost:

Personal Emergency Response Systems may be covered for individuals enrolled in the Medicaid Community Options Entry System. (See previous section for more on COPES).

If you're paying for the service yourself, the monthly fees vary (ranging from $25 to $40), and there are activation charges.

Installation and monitoring fees may apply (unless you are receiving the service through a publicly-funded source).

Examples of businesses that sell medical alert systems:

ADT Companion Service:
☎   **1-800-209-7599**
💻   www.adt.com

Lifeline:
☎   **1-800-380-3111**
💻   www.lifelinesys.com

Link-to-Life:
☎   **1-888-337-5433**
💻   www.link-to-life.com

Telephone Reassurance

Many communities have a program to reassure persons living alone that they will be contacted daily.

Some of these programs are volunteer-based and others are automated calling systems that ask you to respond if you are okay or to request emergency or non emergency help if you need it.

Who to Contact: Call your local Area Agency on Aging (AAA) to find out if a telephone reassurance program is offered in your area. Look in the directory of this guide, under

HELP IN THE COMMUNITY

State Government, for the number of the AAA nearest you.

NOTE: The response time of telephone reassurance is limited to the availability and response of the personal contacts you have pre-selected (such as friends, neighbors, relatives). **Telephone reassurance is not for life-threatening emergencies. It is a safety net. In the event of an emergency, call 9-1-1.**

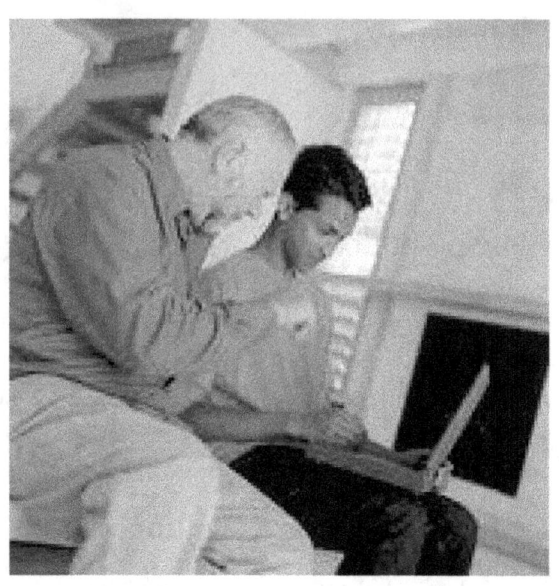

Guardian Calls is an example of a statewide, computerized monitoring service that makes one to six pre-recorded, pre-scheduled calls to make sure you're okay. The fee for either service is $20.00 per month. No one is refused for the lack of funds.

☎   **1-360-275-9385**

💻   **www.guardiancalls.com**

Volunteer Chore Services

Low-income seniors and people with disabilities who don't qualify for other publicly funded supports may be eligible for Volunteer CHORE services, which include transportation, light housekeeping, and shopping. Services are free.

How to Apply: Call or visit your local Area Agency on Aging.

Additional Community Resources

Senior Centers

Senior centers are designated as community focal points through the Older Americans Act.

Many senior centers are supported by government and local non-profit organizations, while others receive funds from organizations such as the YMCA, United Way and Catholic Charities.

The services they offer may include adult day health, meal and nutrition programs, respite, recreation, and educational classes.

Some services, such as on-site meals, are available to any senior who walks in the door (sliding scale fee applies). Other services are based on eligibility.

Contact your local Area Agency on Aging for the senior center in your area, or look in the Yellow Pages of your phone book, under Senior Citizens' Service Organizations.

Public Libraries

Public libraries provide free internet service, interesting classes and workshops, lectures, books on tape, opportunities to volunteer, and people who know how to find anything and everything (that would be librarians, of course).

Community and Faith Based Organizations

Association of Jewish Family & Children's Services

The Association of Jewish Family & Children Services acts as a telephone bridge to link concerned family members of elderly persons living in distant cities with Jewish Family Service Agencies in the community where their loved one lives.

Located in Seattle and Spokane.

☎   1-800-634-7346

💻   www.ajfca.org

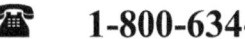

HELP IN THE COMMUNITY

Catholic Charities

Catholic Charities provides social services to individuals in need, including family support, respite care and home care services. Serving people of all faiths. Eligibility varies by program.

💻 **www.catholiccharitiesinfo.org**

Faith in Action

Faith in Action is a network of interfaith volunteer caregiving programs across the country. Volunteers shop, cook, drive or just check in on those with long-term health needs. Eligibility varies by program.

☎ **1-877-324-8411**

💻 **www.fianationalnetwork.org**

Lutheran Services

Lutheran Services provides services ranging from health care to disaster response, as well as care for older adults.

☎ **1-800-664-3848**

💻 **www.lutheranservices.org**

St. Vincent de Paul Society

The St. Vincent de Paul Society provides services ranging from food and nutrition programs, emergency financial assistance, emergency transportation, and homemaker services to anyone in need.

Look in the Yellow Pages of the phone book, under Charities.

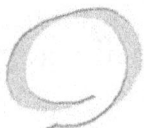

Community Health Programs

Whether you have public or private health insurance, there's always something that's not fully covered.

Community organizations and agencies offer several low-cost and free programs for health services—from discounts on vision care to hearing and eye care.

Community Health Services

The Community Health Services (CHS) program is one of Washington State's primary commitments to ensuring access to primary care for uninsured people.

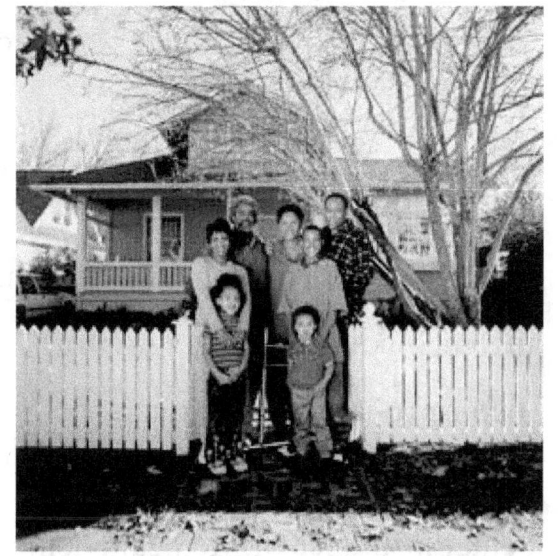

The CHS grant program allocates state dollars to nearly 150 non-profit community health clinics that provide medical and dental care regardless of an individual's ability to pay (sliding fee applies).

For a list of community health clinics in your area, call Community Health Services:

Or visit:

 www.hca.wa.gov/chs/ clinics.html

☎ **360-923-2777**

HELP IN THE COMMUNITY

Dental Care

The Washington State Dental Association (WSDA) Outreach is a discount dental care program for people with disabilities, seniors, elderly, and Alzheimer's patients who are on limited incomes and have no dental insurance or Medicaid dental coupons.

Patients who qualify get a 25 percent discount from participating Washington State Dental Association dentists.

To qualify:

In 2009, patients must have: an annual income under $24,500; a family income (two person or more household) under $33,000; and no dental insurance or Medicaid dental coupons. Seniors must be over age 65, but there is no age limit for Alzheimer's patients or adults with disabilities.

Seniors and people with Alzheimer's: Call your local Area Agency on Aging office (see directory in the back of this guide).

Adults with Disabilities: Call the Washington Oral Health Foundation:

☎   **1-800-448-3368**

☎   **1-206-448-1914**

Eye Care

Seniors EyeCare Program, formerly known as National Eye Care Project (NECP) ensures that every senior has access to medical eye care and promotes annual, dilated eye exams.

Under this program, if you are a U.S. citizen or legal resident age 65 and older, have not seen an ophthalmologist in the last three years or more, and do not belong to an HMO or have Veteran's vision care, you can call for the name of a volunteer ophthalmologist in your area.

Volunteer ophthalmologists will accept Medicare or other insurance as full payment, with no additional payment from you. If you don't have any insurance, the eye care is free.

The ophthalmologist will treat any condition he or she diagnoses during that first visit.

If ongoing care is required for the condition, it will be provided free through this program for one year.

☎   **1-800-222-3937**

SightLife, operated by the Northwest Lions Foundation for Sight and Hearing, provides sight-restoring cornea implants and is one of the leading eye banks in the nation.

☎   **1-800-847-5786**

💻   **www.sightlife.org**

Hearing

Northwest Lions Foundation for Sight and Hearing provides assistance to people with disabilities and low-income for hearing screening and assistive devices on a case-by-case basis.

Northwest Lions Foundation for Sight and Hearing offers a Hearing Aid

Bank for persons with no ability to pay and the AUDIENT program for persons who can participate financially in their hearing care. For information, call:

☎   **1-800-847-5786**

Medical Equipment and Supplies

The correct piece of equipment can mean the difference between isolation and independence, mobility, and an active community life.

Wheelchairs, hospital beds, respiratory equipment, prosthetic and orthotic devices, splints, crutches, trusses, and braces—called Durable Medical Equipment—are examples of supplies covered by Medicare, Medicaid, and private insurance, although coverage and co-pays vary.

Some medical equipment and supply companies offer pharmacy and infusion services, where a nurse administers medication and/or nutritional formulas to patients and

HELP IN THE COMMUNITY

teaches them the proper techniques for self-administration.

Some companies also provide respiratory therapy services to help individuals use breathing equipment.

Insurance plans may require you to use specific suppliers that are under contract with the plan, so be sure to look at the specifics of your plan. In most cases, a prescription is required by your physician.

Check it Out

Some communities have free medical equipment banks from which people can borrow or receive equipment such as wheelchairs, lifts, and walkers.

Check with your local Area Agency on Aging, Independent Living Center, or charitable organizations to find out if such a service exists in your area. (See Directory of Resources.)

Make sure the equipment has been repaired and inspected.

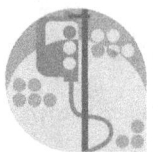

Infusion Therapy

Pharmaceutical and infusion therapy companies specialize in the delivery of drugs, equipment, and professional services for individuals receiving intravenous or nutritional therapies through specially placed tubes.

These companies employ pharmacists who prepare solutions and arrange for delivery to patients.

Nurses also are hired to teach self-administration in patients' homes.

Some pharmaceutical and infusion therapy companies are home health agencies.

Prescription Drugs

Private insurance, Medicare, Medicaid and TRICARE (military health care) all offer prescription drug coverage, although the cost and type of coverage varies.

If you don't have prescription drug coverage, or if what you have is not enough, the following resources can help:

The Washington State Prescription Drug Discount Card is for individuals whose insurance does not cover all their prescription drug needs. There are no other eligibility requirements or fees required for membership in the WPDP. (Note: enrolling in a Medicare Part D plan does **not** disqualify you from enrolling in this program).

On average you'll save up to 60% on generic drugs and 20% on brand name drugs.

✿ Any Washington State resident is eligible for the card.

✿ The card can be used at participating retail pharmacies.

✿ Mail Order and Specialty services are available.

☎   1-800-913-4146

🖥   www.rx.wa.gov

Statewide Health Insurance Benefits Advisors (SHIBA)

The Statewide Health Insurance Benefits Advisors (SHIBA) Helpline provides free health insurance education, assistance and advocacy for all Washington residents.

SHIBA advisors are friendly, knowledgeable and can help you resolve your prescription dilemmas.

☎   1-800-562-6900

☎   1-360-586-0241(TDD)

🖥   **www.insurance.wa.gov**

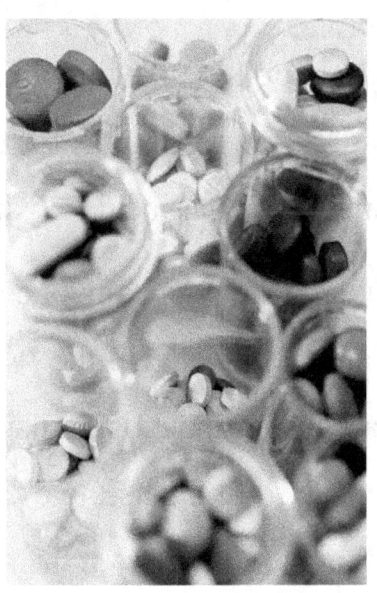

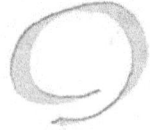

Transportation Options

Transportation options for seniors and people with disabilities vary tremendously from town to town.

Depending on where you live, you may have multiple public transportation options or none at all.

Your best resource for learning about public transportation in your area is your **local transit agency** (such as Spokane Transit or King County Metro).

📖   Look in the yellow pages (under Transportation) for the phone number of your local transit agency.

If you're helping someone who lives in another area, visit the Washington State Department of Transportation website to find a listing of all transit authorities throughout the state:

💻   **www.wsdot.wa.gov**

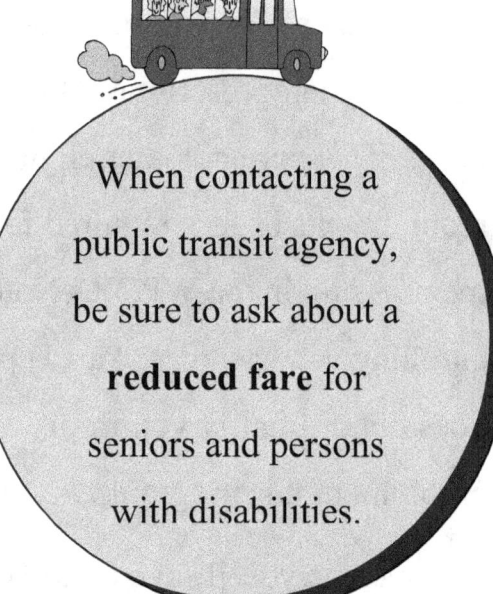

When contacting a public transit agency, be sure to ask about a **reduced fare** for seniors and persons with disabilities.

Door-to-Door (Paratransit)

Door-to-door van service exists within each public transit agency. Service areas are generally related to fixed routes (which means the vans do not cover all areas, only those in which there is a corresponding bus route). Riders must meet eligibility standards. Fares can be paid in exact change or by using a monthly (or annual) pass.

Medicab or Cabulance

Private companies in larger metropolitan areas provide accessible door-to-door transportation for people with disabilities.

The advantage of scheduling a ride through one of these companies is that you can go anywhere in their service area and are not linked to a fixed route bus service. The downside is that they are very costly.

Medical Transportation

The Washington State Department of Social and Health Services (DSHS) pays for transportation services to get to and from needed non-emergency healthcare appointments for persons eligible to receive Medicaid.

If you have a current Medical Assistance Identification Card that is used to pay for your healthcare services and you have no other way to get to your health care appointment,

you may be eligible for transportation.

To request non-emergency medical transportation, contact the contracted agency (called a Regional Broker) that covers the area where you live. Your Regional Broker will arrange the most appropriate, least costly transportation for you.

To find the contracted transportation provider(s) in your area, call the **Medical Assistance Helpline:**

☎ **1-800-562-3022**

☎ **1-800-848-5429 (TTY/TDD)**

(**NOTE:** The best time to call the Medical Assistance Hotline is early in the morning—between 7:00 a.m. and 8:00 a.m. or late in the day—between 5:00 p.m. and 6:00 p.m.—when there's less of a wait.)

Or, visit:

http://fortress.wa.gov/dshs/maa/Transportation/NewPhone.htm

Or, contact your local Area Agency on Aging (see Government Directory).

HELP IN THE COMMUNITY

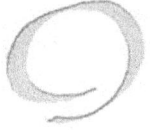

Housing
and Utilities

Affordable Housing

Affordable housing is defined as a home that takes no more than 30 percent of the household's income for rent or mortgage and utilities.

The U.S. Department of Housing and Urban Development (HUD) administers Federal aid to local Public Housing Agencies (PHAs) that manage the housing for low-income residents at rents they can afford. Rent payments are usually based on a percentage of your income.

The following information describes two housing assistance programs managed by local housing agencies:

Housing Choice Vouchers
(Tenant Based)

The housing choice voucher program is the federal government's major program for helping families with very low-income, the elderly, and people with disabilities afford housing in the private market.

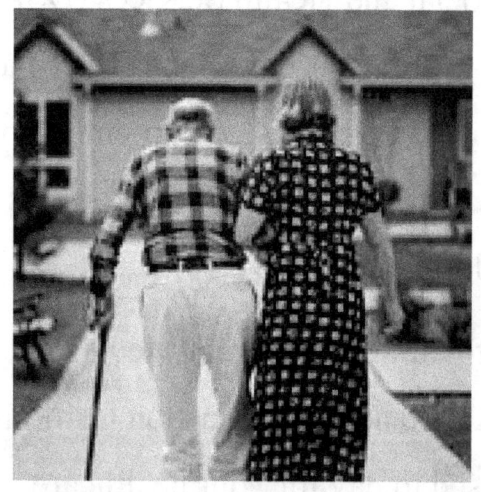

As a tenant-based program, the participant is free to choose any housing that meets the requirements of the program. Its use is not limited to units located in subsidized housing projects.

Local Public Housing Agencies (PHAs) assess eligibility for vouchers. Individuals who are issued a housing voucher by a PHA are responsible for finding a suitable housing unit of their choice where the owner agrees to rent under the program.

This unit may include the individual's present residence. Rental units must meet minimum standards of health and safety, as determined by the public housing agency.

A housing subsidy is paid to the landlord directly by the PHA on behalf of the individual(s).

The individual(s) then pays the difference between the actual rent charged by the landlord and the amount subsidized by the program.

Senior and Disability (Project Based)

Project based rental assistance is attached to the rental unit and does not follow the individual(s) if they move from the assisted unit.

In some cases the housing assistance may be administered by the housing agency or by privately owned and operated properties that manage their own applications and wait lists.

The subsidized properties are divided into two groups:

✿ Family Units

✿ Senior/Elderly and Disability Units

Ask your local housing agency for a list of all project-based properties.

To apply for Rental Assistance, visit your local Public Housing Agency (PHA).

For the office nearest you, look in the Yellow Pages, under Housing Authorities.

Or, call the US Department of Housing and Urban Development Information and Resource Center.

☎   **1-800-955-2232**

HELP IN THE COMMUNITY

Housing Counselors

HUD funds housing counseling agencies throughout the country that give advice free or at low cost.

☎ **1-800-569-4287**

Energy Assistance & Weatherization

The Low Income Home Energy Assistance Program (LIHEAP) is a federally funded program that provides money to help low income households make home heating more affordable, avoid shutoff of utility services during the winter, and maintain a warm, safe, and healthy environment for households with young children, seniors, and people with disabilities.

Payments are made to energy companies in most cases or directly to clients to help pay a portion of home heating costs. Client education and furnace repair/replacement are also offered.

The benefit amount ranges from 50%

to 90% of actual heating costs.

(Source: Department of Community Trade and Economic Development Low Income Home Energy Assistance Program).

Home Weatherization

A statewide network of local community-based nonprofit organizations, known as Community Action Programs (or Councils) provide energy and weatherization services through a grant program.

Weatherization services include: ceiling, wall and floor insulation; closing heat-escaping gaps by caulking, weather stripping, or broken window replacement; and heating system improvements.

☎ **1-360-725-2905**

💻 **www.liheapwa.org**

Home Modification

Home modification includes adaptations to homes that can make it easier and safer for you to live in your own home—such as wheelchair ramps, grab bars, and non-skid strips.

Medicare does not cover home modifications, but Medicaid may cover the cost under programs such as the Community Options Program Entry System (COPES), or a Home and Community Based Waiver

through the Division of Developmental Disabilities (DDD).

If you have the money, and insurance won't cover home modifications, it's well worth the investment to improve the accessibility and safety of your home.

HOME MODIFICATIONS CHECK LIST

Indicators of the Need:

✿ Difficulty getting in and out of the shower

✿ Slipping in the tub or shower

✿ Difficulty turning faucet handles/doorknobs

✿ Access to home

✿ Inadequate heating or ventilation

✿ Problems climbing stairs

Possible Solutions:

✿ Install grab bars, or transfer benches

✿ Use non-skid strips or decals

✿ Replace knobs with lever handles

✿ Install ramps

✿ Install insulation, storm windows and AC

✿ Install handrails for support

Telephone Assistance

The Washington Telephone Assistance Program (WTAP) provides assistance to low-income households, including many senior citizens, who

are without telephones.

Cost: Basic local phone service is $8 a month plus taxes and fees (2008 fee). WTAP pays for only one local phone line per household.

Stand-alone Voicemail - For people who cannot get local phone service, WTAP also provides a voice mailbox service.

Eligibility: You qualify for WTAP if you receive cash, food or medical assistance from the Department of Social and Health Services (DSHS). For more information, call:

☎   **1-888-700-8880**

-OR-

Contact your local telephone company to apply for assistance.

Tribal Lifeline and Link-Up Programs

If you live on a federally recognized reservation, you may be able to save even more money on your phone bill through the federal Tribal Lifeline and Link-Up programs.

How to Apply: Call your local phone company to apply for these enhanced discounts.

HELP IN THE COMMUNITY

TAKING CARE of BUSINESS

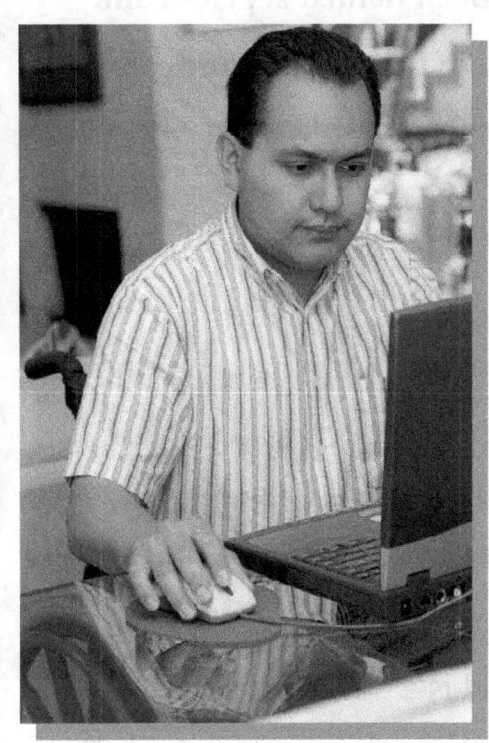

Paying for Services: Don't avoid getting help because of fears about the cost. Learn the basics of health care coverage.

Legal Issues: Powers of Attorney, wills, and guardianships—know your options and protect yourself.

Preventing Abuse and Neglect: Learn the signs. Know what to do if you suspect that someone you know is being harmed.

If You Need to Move Out of Your Home: Learn more about out-of-home residential services and how to find them.

TAKING CARE OF BUSINESS

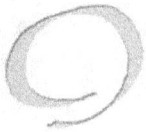

Paying for Services

When it comes to covering the cost of services and supports outlined in this guide, you can either pay for care yourself (private pay) or through health plans (government or private insurance). In many cases, it will be both.

The following chapter provides an overview of the following types of medical coverage:

- Medicaid
- Medicare
- Medicare Savings Program
- Medigap Coverage
- Military and Veterans Benefits
- Healthcare for Workers with Disabilities

NOTE: Eligibility and income requirements are subject to change, so be sure to contact the appropriate resource listed for each type of

coverage for the most up-to-date information.

[See page 66 for legal resources if you've been denied services and would like to appeal that decision.]

TIP: The Statewide Health Insurance Benefits Advisors (SHIBA) HelpLine provides free help to people of all ages with questions about health insurance, health care access, and prescription access: **1-800-562-6900.**

Medicaid

Medicaid is a government health insurance program available to people with limited income and resources. Medicaid does not give you money; rather, it sends payments directly to your health care providers.

Medicaid can pay for medical services in your own home or if you live in a

TAKING CARE OF BUSINESS

residential care facility that takes Medicaid residents.

It covers most of the services outlined in this guide, and is the only publicly funded health care program that pays for long term care (Medicare does not).

There are three different types of Medicaid coverage, depending on your income and resources:

1. Categorically Needy (CN)

2. Medically Needy (MN)

3. Medically Needy with Spend-down

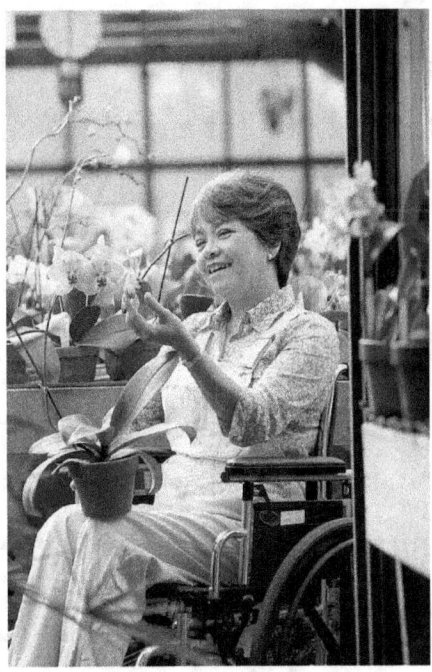

NOTE: Depending on your need for long-term care, the following income guidelines may not necessarily apply.

More liberal income and resource are available to qualify for Medicaid if you meet the standards for needing long-term care services.

As always, contact the appropriate agency (HCS or DDD) to determine your eligibility for Medicaid services.

Categorically Needy (CN)

If you are age 65 or over, blind or have a disability, you may be eligible for Categorically Needy (CN) coverage if your countable income and resource standards are the same or lower than the standards for Supplemental Security Income (SSI).

For 2009, this income standard is $674 per month for an individual and $1,011 per month for a couple.

The program's resource limits are $2,000 for an individual and $3,000 for couples.

Medically Needy (MN)

If your countable income and/or resources are above SSI standards, you may be eligible for the Medically Needy (MN) program. It provides slightly less medical coverage than CN, and greater financial participation by the individuals receiving services.

The Medically Needy (MN) Medicaid program helps pay medical expenses for certain people who are 65 or older and for certain younger people with disabilities. It is sometimes called the "spend-down" program.

Medically Needy Spend-down

Spend-down is the process through which income in excess of the Federal Benefit Rate (FBR) is applied to the cost of your medical care.

For 2010, the FBR is $674 for an individual and $1,011 for a couple (plus a small disregard of $20 per month)

It works sort of like a medical deductible, where you have to incur

medical expenses equal to the excess amount (spend-down) before medical benefits can be authorized.

Example of how spend-down works: If your countable income is $20 over the limit, your medical expenses for the month must be at least $20 in order to make you income-eligible. The higher your income, the higher your spend-down.

There are some exceptions as to what can be counted as income. If you're unsure, call the Medical Assistance Hotline listed at the end of this section.

The program's resource limits for 2010 are $2,000 for an individual and $3,000 for couples.

There is no restriction on how much income you can have when you apply. But the more income you have, the more medical expense you will have to incur before coverage will start.

DSHS rules allow a certain amount of your income to pay for non-medical expenses such as food and shelter.

And, when it calculates how much of your income to set aside for non-medical expenses, DSHS does not count every dollar of income you receive. It's important to learn what counts and what doesn't.

For more information about your Medicaid coverage, call the Medical Assistance Helpline:

☎ **1-800-562-3022**

☎ **1-800-848-5429 (TTY/TDD)**

How to Apply for Medicaid:

Contact your local Community Services Office (CSO). For the number of the office nearest you, call the Aging and Disabilities Administration Helpline:

☎ **1-800-422-3263**

Estate Recovery

Under estate recovery law, the State may be allowed to recover money spent on services provided under Medicaid.

The State may even place a lien on your home if you enter a nursing facility and are not expected to return to your home.

There are more instances where the State may seek to recover money from your estate, and the law is subject to change.

Estate recovery rules can be complicated. Before taking steps you don't understand, you should get individualized legal advice. (See *Legal Issues* for free legal resources.)

RESOURCES

Medicaid and Long-Term Care Services for Adults is a free booklet published by the Department of Social and Health Services.

To download a free copy, enter the following address in the toolbar of your web browser: **www1.dshs.wa.gov/pdf/Publications/22-619.pdf**

TAKING CARE OF BUSINESS

RESOURCES

Estate Recovery for Medical Services Paid for by the State, published by Washington Lawhelp answers common questions about estate recovery.

💻 **www.washingtonlawhelp.org**

(Click on the link for "Health care assistance" and scroll down to "Estate Recovery for Medical Services Paid for by the State".)

For information about Medicaid programs and your rights, visit Washington Lawhelp:

💻   **www.washingtonlawhelp.org**

Washington Lawhelp is provided as a public service by Northwest Justice Project, Washington State's federally-funded legal aid provider in collaboration with other legal aid providers in the Alliance for Equal Justice and Washington courts.

Medicare

Medicare is health insurance for people age 65 or older, under age 65 with certain disabilities, and any age with End-Stage Renal Disease.

Generally speaking, Medicare doesn't pay for long-term care—such as ongoing in-home support, skilled care or facility-based services.

Under certain conditions (such as services related to a recent hospitalization or illness), it will pay for short-term medically necessary skilled nursing facility or home health care.

Medicare has many parts to it. The information on Medicare coverage described in the following pages comes from *Medicare and You 2010*, published by the Centers for Medicaid and Medicare.

For a free copy, call or visit:

☎ **1-800-MEDICARE**

☎ **1-877-486-2048 (TTY)**

💻 **www.medicare.gov**

Medicare Part A (Hospital Insurance)

Medicare Part A helps cover your inpatient care in hospitals and skilled nursing facilities, as well as home health care and hospice if you meet certain conditions.

How to Enroll: If you get benefits from Social Security or the Railroad Retirement Board (RRB), you will automatically get Part A starting the first day of the month you turn age 65.

If you are under age 65 and have a disability, you will automatically get Part A after you get disability benefits from Social Security or RRB for 24 months.

Your Medicare card will be mailed to you about 3 months before your 65th birthday, or your 25th month of disability benefits.

People with ALS (Amyotrophic Lateral Sclerosis, or Lou Gehrig's disease) automatically get Part A the month their disability benefits begin.

Cost: You usually don't pay a monthly premium for Part A coverage if you or your spouse paid Medicare taxes while working.

Medicare Part B (Medical Insurance)

Part B helps cover medically necessary services, such as doctors' services and outpatient care.

There's a lot that Part B doesn't cover—such as prescription drugs, dental, vision, foot care, hearing care and hearing aides, and "custodial care" (which is a Medicare term for personal care).

If you aren't sure if you have Part B, look at your Medicare card. If you

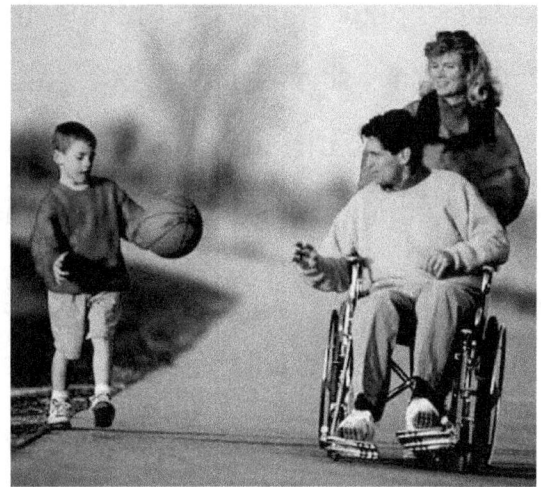

have Part B, "MEDICAL (PART B)" is printed on your card.

Cost: The monthly premium for Part B is $96.40 (2010).

However, your monthly premium will be higher if you are single (file an individual tax return) and your yearly income is more than $85,000, or if you are married (file a joint tax return) and your yearly income is more than $170,000 (2009).

You also pay a Part B deductible each year before Medicare starts to pay its share. In 2010, the deductible amount is $155.

Costs for Part B services vary depending on the type of service you get and the type of plan you choose.

To Apply: Call the Social Security Administration (SSA):

☎ **1-800-772-1213**

☎ **1-800-325-0778 (TTY)**

Saving on Your Part B Premium
There are two ways to save on your Part B premium:

1) A few Medicare Advantage Plans may pay all or part of your Part B premium. You still get all Part A and Part B-covered services.

2) You can also call your State Medical Assistance (Medicaid) office to see if you can get help paying your Part B premium costs.

Medicare Part C (Medicare Advantage Plans)

Part C (also known as Medicare Advantage Plans) combines Part A, Part B, and sometimes Part D prescription drug coverage.

Medicare Advantage Plans are managed by private insurance companies approved by Medicare.

These plans must cover medically-necessary services. However, plans can charge different co-payments, coinsurance, or deductibles for these services.

Medicare Advantage Plans may offer extra benefits beyond what you would get from Part A and B, such as vision, hearing, dental, and/or health and wellness programs. Most include Medicare prescription drug coverage (for an extra cost).

Cost: You will generally still pay the monthly Part B premium, plus the Medicare Advantage Plan's premium (if they charge one), which includes coverage for Part A and Part B benefits, prescription drug coverage and any other extra benefits.

To learn more about costs:

☎ **1-800-MEDICARE**

☎ **1-877-486-2048 (TTY)**

-OR-

💻 **www.medicare.gov**

Medicare Part D (Prescription Drug Coverage)

Medicare offers prescription drug coverage for everyone with Medicare through Part D, which is an optional plan with a monthly premium.

To get Medicare drug coverage, you must join a Medicare drug plan run by insurance companies and other private companies approved by Medicare.

Each plan varies in cost and drugs covered.

If you decide not to join a Medicare drug plan when you are first eligible, you may pay a late-enrollment penalty if you choose to join later.

There are two ways to get Medicare prescription drug coverage:

1) Join a Medicare Prescription Drug Plan. These plans (sometimes called "PDPs") add drug coverage to the Original Medicare Plan, some Medicare Cost Plans, some Medicare Private Fee-for-Service (PFFS) Plans, and Medicare Medical Savings Account (MSA) Plans.

2) Join a Medicare Advantage Plan (Part C) or another Medicare health plan that includes prescription drug coverage.

You get all of your Medicare coverage (Part A and Part B), including prescription drugs (Part D), through these plans. These plans are sometimes called "MA-PD's."

Both types of plans are called "Medicare drug plans" in this section.

If you join a Medicare drug plan, you usually pay a separate monthly premium in addition to your Part B premium.

Cost: Monthly premium (varies by plan); yearly deductible; co-payments or coinsurance.

Medigap (Medicare Supplement Insurance)

Since Medicare Part A and B pays for many, but not all, health care services and supplies, another option is to consider buying a Medigap policy sold by private insurance companies.

A Medigap policy is private health insurance designed to supplement the Original Medicare Plan (Parts A and B).

This means it helps pay some of the health care costs ("gaps") that the Original Medicare Plan doesn't cover, like copayments, coinsurance, and deductibles.

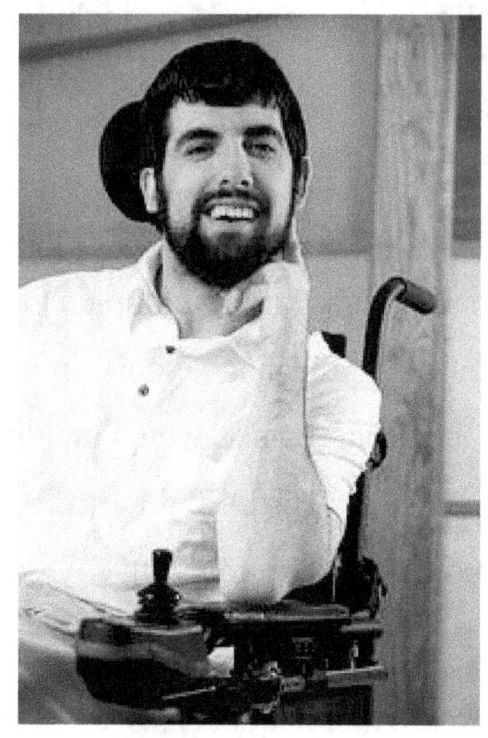

Some Medigap policies cover extra benefits for an extra cost. If you are in the Original Medicare Plan and you buy a Medigap policy, then both plans will pay their share of Medicare-approved amounts for covered health care costs.

Medigap policies only work with the Original Medicare Plan, and they can't be used to pay your co-payments or deductibles for Medicare Advantage Plans.

They must follow Federal and state laws designed to protect you. Every

Medigap policy must be clearly identified as Medicare Supplement Insurance.

Each standardized Medigap policy must offer the same basic benefits, no matter which insurance company sells it.

Usually the only difference between Medigap policies is the cost.

Medicare Savings Programs

If you need help paying for all or part of your Medicare premiums, and you meet income and resource requirements, you may be able to get help from a Medicare Savings Program.

There are three Medicare Savings Programs available:

1) Qualified Medicare Beneficiary Program (QMB)

2) Specified Low-Income Medicare Beneficiary Program (SLMB)

3) Qualified Individual(QI-1) Program

The following income limits are provided as a guideline. People with gross income above these levels— particularly when earnings are involved—may still qualify. Check your eligibility by applying.

For any of the cost-sharing programs your resources (assets) must be under $6,600 for an individual and $9,910 for a couple (2010).

Income limits are different in each program and listed under the program information.

Qualified Medicare Beneficiary (QMB) Program:

QMB pays your Part B Medicare premium, and the cost, if any, of your Part A premium.

QMB also pays your Medicare co-payments and deductibles.

To be eligible your income must be no more than:

- $903.00 per month for one person (2010); or

- $1,215.00 per month for a couple (2010)

Special Low-Income Medicare Beneficiary (SLMB):

You must be eligible for or be enrolled in Medicare Part A. Income limits are over 100 percent of the Federal Poverty Level (FPL) but under 120 percent of the FPL.

Under SLMB, DSHS will pay your Medicare Part B premium only.

Monthly income limit:

- $1,083.00 per month for one person (2010); or

- $1,457.00 per month for a couple (2010)

Qualified Individual (QI-1) Program:

You must be eligible for or enrolled in Medicare Part A and not eligible for

any other Medicaid coverage.

Monthly income limit:

- $1,219 per month for one person (2010); or

- $1,640 per month for a couple (2010)

Additional information on Medicare Savings Programs is available at the Health and Recovery Services Administration website:

⌨   **www.dshs.wa.gov/pdf/Publications/22-500.pdf**

How to apply:

Contact your local Community Services Office (CSO). For the location of the CSO nearest you, call the Aging and Disability Services Administration Helpline:

☎   **1-800-422-3263**

Medicare Has You Covered

From *Stay Active and Independent for Life: An Information Guide for Adults 65+*, published by the Washington State Department of Health

Medicare can help you with your goals of staying active and independent. At the time of this publication, Medicare coverage includes:

- **Professional treatment of foot problems and foot care** for diabetes and other medical conditions.

- **Therapeutic footwear and inserts** (orthotics), if prescribed by a doctor.

- **Assistive devices**, covered with a doctor's prescription by Medicare Part B under the Original Medicare Plan.

- **Vision screening and care** by an ophthalmologist or optometrist.

- **Hearing screening and care** by an ear, nose, and throat doctor or licensed audiologist.

- **Bone density tests** every two years to diagnose or monitor osteoporosis.

- **Osteoporosis screening** by a primary care, family practice, or internal medicine physician, or a rheumatologist.

- An **orthopedic surgeon** for muscle, ligament, tendon, bone, joint problems.

- A **rheumatologist** for joint pain in two or more different joints or unexplained muscle pain.

- A **neurologist** for balance problems, for balance problems, dizziness.

- A **physical therapist** for walking problems, muscle or joint problems, and walker and cane training.

- An **occupational therapist** for assistive devices to help with daily activities.

TAKING CARE OF BUSINESS

Veterans Benefits

If you are a veteran or have served in the U.S. military, contact the U.S. Department of Veterans Affairs (VA) for information about veterans' benefits and services available in your area:

☎ **1-800-827-1000**

💻 **www.va.gov**

Veterans in Washington State that use Medicaid to pay for long-term care services can get help tracking down benefits. For more information, call the DSHS Veterans Project:

☎ **1-800-280-0586**

Military Benefits (TRICARE)

TRICARE is a health care program for active-duty service members, retirees, and their families. The uniformed services determine who is eligible for TRICARE coverage. All people with TRICARE are eligible for TRICARE pharmacy benefits. You may also add Medicare prescription drug coverage. For more information, contact TRICARE:

☎ **1-866-773-0404**

💻 **www.tricare.osd.mil**

Healthcare for Workers with Disabilities (HWD)

Healthcare for Workers with Disabilities is a Categorically Needy medical program that recognizes the employment potential of people with disabilities.

Under this program, people with disabilities (age 16 through 64) can earn more money and purchase healthcare coverage for an amount based on a sliding income scale.

Healthcare for Workers with Disabilities has no asset test and the income limits are based on 220 percent of the Federal Poverty level (FPL).

Effective April 1, 2009 the monthly income limit is:

$1,986 for one person

$2,672 for two people

To be eligible, a person must meet federal disability requirements, be employed (including self-employment) full or part time and pay a monthly premium.

Cost: Based on a sliding scale, not to exceed 7.5% of your total income.

To Apply: Call 1-800-337-1835, choose option 2 for "family or adult medical" and tell the Customer Service Specialist that you are calling about HWD.

Note: If you receive services through Home and Community Services or DDD, contact your case manager for assistance.

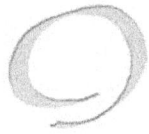

Legal Issues

Note: The following information is not a substitute for legal advice. Specific questions about your situation should be addressed with an attorney.

Regardless of your age or disability, it's important that you have a say in decisions made about your life.

One way to protect your rights is to make sure you have legal documents specifying what you want to happen if you lose the ability to make decisions for yourself.

Without these documents, someone else can seek to represent your interests through guardianship if it can be shown that you are unable to handle your own affairs.

There are alternatives to guardianship that you can take while you're able to make your wishes clear.

These options may be worth pursuing, as long you understand the intent and effect of the document you are signing.

Financial Decisions

Power of Attorney

A *power of attorney* gives someone else (known as the *agent* or *attorney-in-fact*) legal authority to act for you (the *principal*) on your behalf.

A Power of Attorney (POW) document defines the powers that the agent is authorized to perform.

This can include management of all or part of your finances, including:

✿ buying and selling

✿ cashing checks

✿ managing a business

✿ investing money

✿ general management of finances

POW's may also include the management of personal affairs, and/or health care decisions (you can

---

also create a power of attorney for health care only, see section on Health Decisions).

Both you and the person you select as your agent have these powers.

TIP:

Granting someone powers of attorney does not mean that you lose the ability to sign and manage your own affairs. If you can easily make the decision yourself, try to maintain control over how and when a power of attorney is used.

A power of attorney without a "durable provision" (see following definition) will become ineffective if you become incapacitated due to disability.

It can continue (or even begin) when you become incapacitated if you include a "durable provision."

A provision for *durable power of attorney* includes language indicating that the power will continue in the event of incapacitation or disability.

FIVE WISHES

Five Wishes, created by Aging with Dignity, lets your family and doctors know:

1. Which person you want to make health care decisions for you when you can't make them.

2. The kind of medical treatment you want or don't want.

3. How comfortable you want to be.

4. How you want people to treat you.

5. What you want your loved ones to know.

For more information about Five Wishes, and to obtain a copy, visit:

💻 www.agingwithdignity.org

If the document lacks this kind of language, the power of attorney is not "durable," and it terminates if you become unable to manage your affairs.

A durable power of attorney may be written to take effect immediately or to take effect only if you become incapacitated.

The latter type of power of attorney is called a ***springing durable power of attorney***.

These powers of attorney should include language describing how incapacity will be determined.

Durable powers of attorney are relatively simple and inexpensive to arrange compared to trusts or guardianships.

NOTE: Allowing someone else to handle your finances has the potential to allow financial exploitation.

Ensure that the person managing your affairs is:

o   Trustworthy

o   Stable

o   Available

It's important to talk to the person you want to appoint and make sure he/she understands what you want and will follow your wishes.

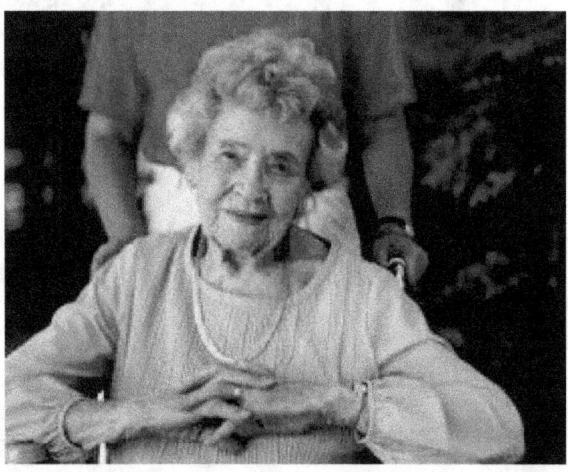

Powers of attorney are not recognized by the Social Security Administration (SSA).

Instead, SSA requires a ***representative payee***, who is someone authorized by SSA to receive and manage the government benefits on behalf of a person determined incapacitated by disability.

There is little oversight of the representative payee system. Misuse of funds may go unnoticed or unreported. If this is the case with you or someone you know, contact Adult Protective Services:

1-866-363-4276

Trusts

A trust is a legal arrangement through which property or money is held by one person (the *trustee*) to benefit another (the *beneficiary*).

Trusts are flexible tools that can accommodate a variety of goals; however, they are complex, and require careful consideration, drafting, and management.

Trusts might not make practical sense for a person with small assets. Advice of an attorney specializing in trusts is important.

Trusts can affect Medicaid eligibility or have tax consequences. An exception to this is a ***special needs trust***.

Special needs trusts are frequently used to receive an inheritance or personal injury settlement proceeds on behalf of someone with a disability or are founded from the proceeds of compensation for criminal injuries, litigation or insurance settlements.

Health Care Decisions

Durable Power of Attorney for Health Care Decisions

A *durable health care power of attorney* can give someone you appoint (your *agent*) the authority to make health care decisions on your behalf if you become unable to make such decisions.

Many durable power of attorney forms DO NOT include authority for health care decisions. Some people choose to have one durable power of attorney for health decisions and a separate durable power of attorney for financial decisions.

If you chose to have a durable power of attorney for health care decisions, make sure the person you name as your agent knows you well enough to make the kind of decisions you would make for yourself.

You can create a document that makes your agent's power as limited or general as you wish. Just like a financial power of attorney, a health

TAKING CARE OF BUSINESS

TAKING CARE OF BUSINESS

care power of attorney is no longer in effect if you become incapacitated unless you include durable provisions.

Wills

A will is a legal document that outlines what happens to your property after you die.

It defines who is to get the property and in what amounts. If necessary, a will can also

- name a guardian for any minor children (or pets);
- identify someone else to handle the property left after death on behalf of children or others; and/or,
- identify an "executor" to handle property and affairs from the time of death until an estate is settled.

Learn more about wills from the Washington Bar Association website: www.wsba.org/media/publications/pamphlets/wills.htm

Living Will or Health Care Directive

A living will is a legal document that defines for health care professionals what type, if any, of medical treatments you want to prolong your life if an accident or undiagnosed life threatening illness occurs and you are unable to communicate your wishes.

A living will only comes into effect when you are near death. The Washington State Department of Health offers a free on-line registry that lets Washington State residents have their end-of-life preferences available online to authorized health care providers.

Visit the Washington State Living Will Registry for more information:

⌨ **www.doh.wa.gov/livingwill**

Physician Orders for Life-Sustaining Treatment (POLST) or Do Not Resuscitate (DNR)

A Physician Orders for Life-Sustaining Treatment (POLST) form allows you to document what, if any, medical treatments you want to prolong your life if you are currently terminally ill.

Your doctor has an end-of life discussion with you and translates your wishes into actual physician's orders on the POLST form.

Having a completed POLST form helps make sure your wishes are followed by other medical professionals without delay.

The POLST form must be an original and not a copy. Learn more about POLST from the Washington State Medical Association:

🖥 **www.wsma.org/patients/polst**

Guardianship

If you become incapacitated and you have not established a durable power of attorney for financial and health decisions (or the provisions you made will not meet your needs), someone (such as a family member, friend, care facility, or case manager) may petition the court to appoint a legal guardian for you.

Guardianships can be costly and time consuming. They also seriously compromise your personal autonomy.

The court can appoint a guardian for the *person*, the *person's financial estate*, or both. A guardian for the person can be appointed if the court determines you to be at risk of personal harm based on your inability to adequately provide food, health, housing, or physical safety.

A guardian of the estate can be appointed when the court determines that you are at risk of financial harm based on an inability to manage your financial affairs.

Guardianships can be full or limited.

A full guardianship covers all decisions allowed by law for someone who is incapacitated.

A limited guardianship specifies certain areas where the guardian can make decisions, allowing the individual to make all other decisions for him/herself.

TAKING CARE OF BUSINESS

TAKING CARE OF BUSINESS

Legal Resources

Coordinated Legal Education, Advice and Referral System (CLEAR, CLEAR*Sr)

CLEAR provides free legal assistance to low-income people with civil legal problems.

Clear Sr is available to persons age 60 and older without regard to income.

Interpreter services are available.

Inside King County:

☎   1-206-464-1519

Outside King County:

☎   1-888-201-1014

CLEAR*Sr (for people over 60)

☎   1-888-387-7111

☎   1-888-201-9737 (TTY)

💻   **www.nwjustice.org**

Disability Rights Washington

A nonprofit organization providing legal advocacy services to Washington residents with disabilities. Services include: Information and referral; Legal representation; Abuse or neglect investigation. Serves all people with disabilities.

☎   **1-800-562-2702**

☎   **1-800-905-0209 (TTY)**

Interpreters available in over 200 languages via AT&T Language Line.

💻   **www.disabilityrightswa.org**

Caring Connections

Caring Connections, a program of the National Hospice and Palliative Care Organization, is a national initiative to improve care at the end of life, supported by a grant from The Robert Wood Johnson Foundation.

Caring Connections provides free resources and information to help people make decisions about end-of-life care and services before a crisis.

☎   **1-800-658-8898**

Cuidando con Cariño:

☎   **1-877-658-8896**

Bi-lingual staff are available to assist callers with end-of-life care issues.

Dispute Resolution Centers Elder Mediation Program

The Elder Mediation Program within Dispute Resolution Centers assist elders, their families and caregivers with resolving conflict that may arise around issues of autonomy, housing, health care or end-of-life decisions.

Trained mediators will meet with families throughout the region. No one is turned away due to lack of funds.

🖥️   **www.resolutionwa.org**

National Academy of Elder Law Attorneys (NAELA)

An online directory of attorneys who deal with legal issues affecting seniors and persons with disabilities.

🖥️   **www.naela.com**

National Association of County Veteran Service Officers (NACVSO)

NACVSO provides assistance in obtaining veterans' benefits and answers questions regarding rules and regulations concerning veterans.

For veterans and family members.

🖥️   **www.nacvso.org**

Washington LawHelp

Washington Lawhelp is provided as a public service by Northwest Justice Project, Washington State's federally-funded legal aid provider in collaboration with other legal aid providers in the Alliance for Equal Justice and Washington courts.

Washington Lawhelp provides more details on many of the issues described in this section—including guardianship, powers of attorney to living wills. For more information, visit:

🖥️ **www.washingtonlawhelp.org**

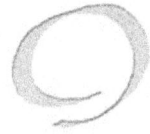

Preventing Abuse and Neglect

Abuse and neglect is a challenging topic for many people to deal with. But the more it's ignored, the more chance it has to take root in your life or the life of someone you know.

According to the National Center on Elder Abuse, "It has been estimated that roughly two-thirds of those who harm vulnerable adults are family members—most often the victim's adult child or spouse."

For yourself and those you love:

✿ Know the signs of abuse

✿ Report any suspicion of abuse

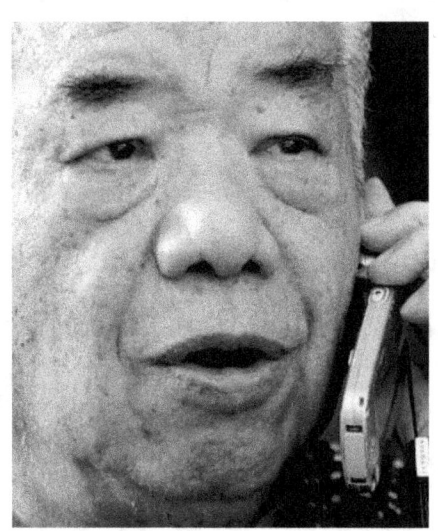

The following pages will help you recognize the signs of abuse and how to report incidents of physical, emotional, psychological or financial harm.

Report Abuse and You May Save a Life

If you suspect abuse or neglect of a vulnerable adult, **call 1-866-ENDHARM. (1-866-363-4276).** Call this one number and you could save a life. A person will answer your call 24 hours a day, seven days a week.

In an emergency situation, call 911.

TAKING CARE OF BUSINESS

Recognize Signs of Abuse

Physical

Slap marks, most pressure marks, unexplained burns or blisters (such as cigarette burns), explanations that don't seem to fit with the pattern of physical injury.

Sexual

Bruises around the breasts or genital area and unexplained sexually transmitted diseases.

Mental/Emotional

Withdrawal from normal activities, nervousness around certain people, agitation, unusual behavior (rocking, biting).

Financial Exploitation

Sudden change in finances and accounts, altered wills and trusts, unusual bank withdrawals, checks written as "loans" or "gifts," and loss of property.

Neglect

Untreated bedsores, need for medical or dental care, unclean clothing, poor hygiene, overgrown hair and nails, and unusual weight loss.

Self Neglect

Refusing medication, alcohol or substance abuse, isolation, unsanitary living conditions (soiled bedding, fleas, feces and urine smell), poor hygiene, malnourished.

Abandonment

Deserting a vulnerable adult in public, or deserting him/her in their own home.

If you have concerns that someone you know is being abused, or neglected, trust your instincts.

Ask questions.

Remember that the victim of abuse may be experiencing other problems and more than one type of abuse.

TAKING CARE OF BUSINESS

Report Abuse

To report abuse or neglect of a vulnerable adult or a child in Washington State, call the DSHS toll-free EndHarm hotline anytime day or night:

Toll-free: 1-866-363-4276

ENDHARM is TTY accessible. When you call, you will speak with a real person, who will connect you to the local number to make your report.

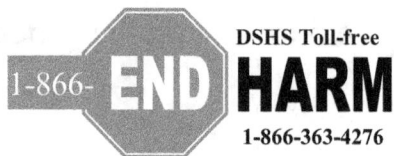

DSHS Toll-free
1-866- END HARM
1-866-363-4276

Protect Yourself from Abuse

✿ Stay busy and engaged in life.

✿ Don't become isolated, and don't allow anyone else to isolate you by not allowing you to talk to other people outside their presence.

✿ Take care of your health—keep your doctor and dental appointments.

✿ If an adult relative wants to live with you, think it over carefully, especially if the individual is having personal problems or a history of violent behavior, drug or alcohol abuse.

✿ Be clear about what you will and will not tolerate and set boundaries.

✿ Trust that little voice inside that tells you when something isn't right.

✿ Seek the advice of a trusted friend, attorney, family member or physician before you act on major decisions and/or purchases.

✿ Maintain a strong support system of family and friends who are concerned about your well-being.

✿ Don't let anyone keep you from the telephone or prevent you from leaving your house.

✿ If you're living with someone else, have your own phone and handle your own mail.

Protect Yourself from Financial Exploitation

Phone Scams

Do not give your credit card information, social security number or bank account numbers over the phone.

Telephone scam artists try to get your personal information by offering prizes, credit cards and other false benefits.

If it seems too good to be true, it usually is.

Finances

Be thoroughly familiar with your financial status and know how to handle your assets.

Organize your financial documents in one place for easy and quick reference.

Do not add another person's name to bank or insurance documents without legal advice.

Consider direct deposit for any regular monthly income.

Hiring Contractors

Get two or more bids for home repair work from reputable contractors. Make sure they are bonded and licensed.

Be careful about having more work done than is needed. It's okay to say "enough!"

Learn if a contractor is currently registered, and whether action against the contractor's bond is pending or has been taken in the past.

Call the Washington State Department of Labor and Industries Contractor Registration Verification to make sure the contractor or person you are hiring is actively licensed, with a current bond and insurance, and an electrician or plumber is certified (licensed) in Washington:

☎   **1-800-647-0982**

Make sure you check the references of any contractor you hire. If possible, perform a background check. Rule out

TAKING CARE OF BUSINESS

anyone with a history of violence, alcohol or drug abuse.

Keep valuables in a safe place.

Legal Issues

Do not sign any document until you or someone you trust has read it.

Get legal advice for questions regarding power of attorney or durable power of attorney. Make sure that the person you designate as your power of attorney is someone you know and trust well.

Be wary about deeding or willing your house or other assets to anyone who promises to keep you out of a nursing home or take care of you at home if you become disabled. This is a common scam.

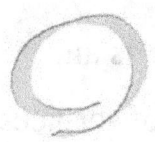

If You Need to Move...

Choosing Out-of-Home Options

Although this guide is designed for people living at home, there may come a time to consider out-of-home options.

If you or someone you know is no longer able to continue living at home, there are several types of facilities that provide care in small to large congregate settings known as *residential care*.

It's important to know that if state funds are being used, the facility must be licensed by Washington State and agree to accept payments by Medicaid.

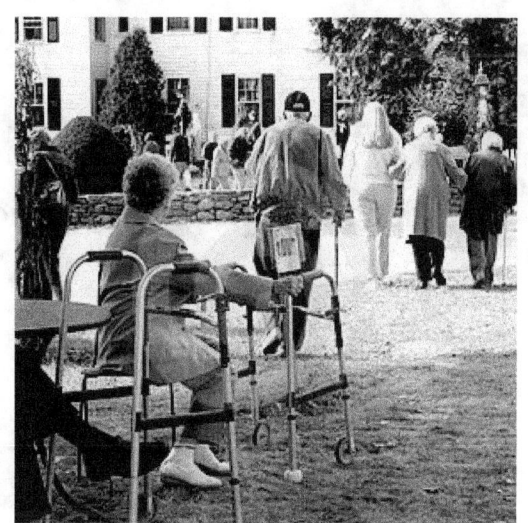

Adult Family Homes

Adult Family Homes are regular neighborhood homes licensed by the state and run by a family, single person, or business partners.

Some specialize in care for people with mental health conditions, developmental disabilities or dementia. The home can have two to six residents.

A room, meals, laundry, supervision and varying levels of assistance with care are provided. Some provide occasional nursing care.

To explore an AFH as an option, find out what kinds of services and

TAKING CARE OF BUSINESS

supports are available at each home you are interested in.

For a list of licensed Adult Family Homes in your area, call the Aging and Disability Services Administration Helpline:

☎   **1-800-422-3263**

-OR-

🖥   **www.adsa.dshs.wa.gov**

(Click on "Assisted Living Options")

Boarding Homes

Boarding Homes are facilities in a community setting with seven or more residents.

Housing, meals, laundry, supervision, and varying levels of assistance with care are provided. Some provide nursing care.

Some offer specialized care for people with mental health issues, developmental disabilities, or dementia.

To explore a boarding home as an option, find out what kinds of services and supports are available at each of the different facilities you are interested in.

Reputation Matters

✿ Ask a representative of the home to show you the last state inspection report. This will show you if there are any issues you need to be aware of.

✿ Ask for references or contact information of former residents or family members.

✿ Ask for a copy of the disclosure form that spells out the care and services offered. (For Boarding Homes Only.)

✿ Contact the DSHS Field Manager in your area to find out about past complaints. For the number of the Field Manager, call the **Aging and Disability Services Administration Helpline:**

☎   **1-800-422-3263**

Once you get a list of local homes,

begin making calls to arrange a visit. It takes time, but it's a necessary part of looking for the right facility and getting a good "feel" for the type of environment you will be living in.

Ask about…

✿ Costs and financing (type of insurance coverage or private pay policies)

✿ Refund policies

✿ Types of services

✿ Flexibility of schedule for receiving personal care

✿ Staff turnover rate

✿ Length of time under the current administration

✿ Language(s) spoken by most staff

For a list of licensed boarding homes in your area contact the Aging and Disability Services Administration:

☎   **1-800-422-3263**

💻   **www.adsa.dshs.wa.gov**

(Click on Assisted Living Options)

Nursing Homes

Skilled nursing facilities (SNF) and nursing facilities (NF) are licensed to care for people who can't be cared for at home or in the community due to complex medical conditions.

Nursing homes provide 24-hour supervised nursing care, personal care, therapy, nutrition management, organized activities, social services, room, board and laundry.

Compare Nursing Homes in Washington State

Concerned about a nursing home's performance? The U.S. Dept of Health and Human Services offers great online information about the past performance of every Medicare and Medicaid certified nursing home in the country.

Visit: **www.medicare.gov** and click on "Compare Home Health Agencies in Your Area."

Short-term Nursing Home Stays

Entering a nursing home doesn't mean you need to stay forever.

You can receive care in a nursing home for rehabilitation or for short-term, intensive nursing care.

If you need short-term nursing home care, plan ahead for the types of services and support you may need after leaving the facility to return home or to another residential care setting.

Call Senior Information and Assistance for help figuring out your options. For the number in your area, see page 105-107 in the Government Directory, or visit:

⌨   **www.adsa.dshs.wa.gov**

(Click on Find Local Services)

To locate a licensed Nursing Home in your area, call the Aging and Disability Services Administration Helpline:

☎   **1-800-422-3263**

Or visit the Aging and Disability Services Administration website:

⌨   **www.adsa.dshs.wa.gov**

(Click on Assisted Living Options)

Continuing Care Retirement Communities (CCRC's)

A Continuing Care Retirement Community (CCRC) is a residential community for adults that offers a range of housing options (independent living through nursing home care) and varying levels of medical and personal care services.

A CCRC is designed to meet a resident's needs in a familiar setting as he/she grows older.

They are not licensed by the State of Washington.

They may require buy-in, or an up-front annuity purchase followed by monthly payments covering services, amenities and needed medical. The buy-in may be refundable in part, or not at all.

In the same community, there may be individual homes or apartments for residents who still live on their own,

an assisted living facility for people who need some help with daily care, and a nursing home for those who require higher levels of care.

Residents move from one level of care to another based on their needs but still stay in the CCRC.

If you are considering a CCRC, be sure to check the record of its nursing home. Your CCRC contract usually requires you to use the CCRC nursing home if you need this level of care.

Many of the questions that you might want to ask about these communities are the same as those to consider when choosing a nursing home.

CCRC's generally charge a large payment before you move in (called an entry fee) and then charge monthly fees.

You can find out if a CCRC is accredited and get advice on selecting

this type of long-term care community from the Commission on Accreditation of Rehabilitation Facilities:

💻 **www.carf.org**

Washington State does not license retirement communities. To find local retirement communities in the area, contact your local Senior Information and Assistance. For the number in your area, see page 105-107 in the Government Directory, or visit:

💻 **www.adsa.dshs.wa.gov**

(Click on Find Local Services)

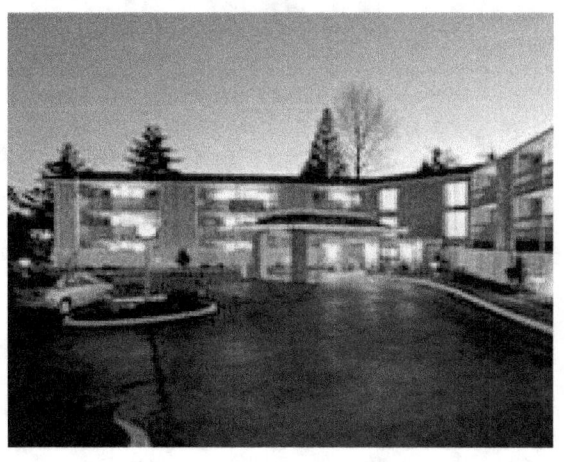

TAKING CARE OF BUSINESS

Senior Housing Locator

Aging and Disability Services Administration offers a free online information resource to help you search for senior housing in Washington State. Search for Assisted living, nursing & rehabilitation homes and Continuing Care Retirement Communities (CCRC's) by geographic location.

www.aasa.dshs.wa.gov/Lookup/BHPubLookup.asp

DIRECTORY

of

RESOURCES*

*Information contained in this directory is subject to change. As of the date of this printing, the phone numbers and websites are accurate.

Topical Directory

-A-

Abuse and Neglect

Adult Protective Services (see Directory of Government Agencies—State and Local)

Complaint Resolution Unit (see Directory of Government Agencies—State and Local)

EndHarm
To report abuse or neglect of a vulnerable adult or a child in Washington State, call the DSHS toll-free EndHarm hotline anytime day or night. ENDHARM is TTY accessible. When you call, you will speak with a real person, who will connect you to the direct local number to make your report:

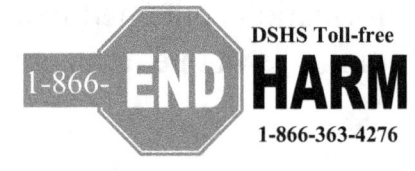

☎   **1-866-363-4276**

Long Term Care Ombudsman
Volunteer Long-Term Care Ombudsmen respond to complaints about Adult Family Homes, Boarding Homes and Nursing Homes.
☎   **1-800-562-6028**

Adult Day Services

Washington Adult Day Services Association
The Washington Adult Day Services Association is a coalition of adult day care and adult day health providers throughout the state of Washington. Call to find out the number of your local Adult Day Services providers.
☎ **1-888-609-2372**
🖥 **www.adultday.org**

Alzheimer's Disease

Alzheimer's Association
Provides reliable information, care consultation and supportive services for dementia caregivers through state and local chapters. The website also includes an interactive tool, CareFinder, which helps families to recognize quality dementia care; plan and pay for care; communicate with care providers; and find local support and resources.
☎ **1-800-272-3900** (24 hours 7 days a week)
🖥 **www.alz.org**

Alzheimer's Disease Education and Referral (ADEAR) Center
Information and resources for health professionals, people with Alzheimer's disease and their families, and the public.
☎ **1-800-438-4380** (8:30 a.m. to 5:00 p.m. Eastern Time, Monday - Friday)
🖥 **www.alzheimers.org/index.html**

Alzheimer's Resource Room
The Alzheimer's Resource Room is an online resource for families, caregivers, and professionals.
🖥 **www.answersforfamilies.org**

Arthritis

Arthritis Foundation
With 46 local offices around the country, the Arthritis Foundation offers many resources for a variety of services. Call for local Arthritis Foundation offices and resources.
☎ **1-800-283-7800**
🖥 **www.arthritis.org**

Cancer

CancerCare
CancerCare is a national nonprofit organization that provides free, professional support services for anyone affected by cancer.
☎ **1-800-813-HOPE (4673)**
🖥 **www.cancercare.org**

DIRECTORY—TOPICAL

Caregiver Support

Children of Aging Parents
A nonprofit membership organization that provides information and referral services for a variety of professionals, information about support groups, and educational outreach services.
🖳 **www.caps4caregivers.org**

Caring From a Distance
Caring From a Distance is a nonprofit organization created by men and women dealing with long distance care.
🖳 **www.cfad.org**

Family Care Navigator
State-by-State Help for Family Caregivers.
🖳 **www.caregiver.org**

-D-

Dental Care

The Washington State Dental Association (WSDA) Outreach is a discount dental care program for people with disabilities, seniors, elderly, and Alzheimer's patients who are on limited incomes and have no dental insurance or Medicaid dental coupons. Patients who qualify get a 25 % discount from participating Washington State Dental Association dentists.
Seniors and people with Alzheimer's disease: Please call your local Area Agencies on Aging office.
Adults with Disabilities: Please call the Washington Oral Health Foundation:
☎ **1-800-448-3368; 1-206-448-1914**

Diabetes

The American Diabetes Association
The American Diabetes Association funds research and provides information and other services to people with diabetes, their families, health professionals and the public.
🖳 **www.diabetes.org**

Defeat Diabetes Foundation
The Defeat Diabetes Foundation is a non-profit organization that provides information to people with diabetes, pre-diabetes and the public.
💻 **www.DefeatDiabetes.org**

Disability—Traumatic Brain Injury

Brain Injury Association of Washington
The Brain Injury Association of Washington provides support to survivors of brain injury and their families, education to those who are being affected by brain injury, including the general public, and advocacy.
☎ **Helpline: 1-866-982-4292**
TBI Washington Information and Referral Line:
☎ **1-877-TBI-1766 (1-877-824-1766)** In case of technical difficulties,
☎ call: **425-778-3707**
💻 **www.tbiwashington.org**
💻 **www.biawa.org**

Defense and Veterans Brain Injury Center (DVBIC)
The Defense and Veterans Brain Injury Center (DVBIC) serves active duty military, their dependents and veterans with traumatic brain injury (TBI) through state-of-the-art medical care, innovative clinical research initiatives and educational programs.
💻 **www.dvbic.org**

☎ **1-800-870-9244**

☎ **1-202-556-6809**

Disability Rights Washington (see Topical Directory—Legal)

Disability—Developmental

The Arc of Washington State
The Arc of Washington State is a non-profit organization that provides information and systems advocacy on behalf of children and adults with developmental disabilities.
☎ **1-888-754-8798**; 💻 **www.arcwa.org**

Local Arc Chapters

☎ **The Arc of Clark County**
360-254-1562 (Ext. 17); 🖥 **www.arcofclarkcounty.org**

☎ **The Arc of Cowlitz Valley**
360-425-5494; 🖥 www.cowlitzarc.org

☎ **The Arc of Grays Harbor**
360- 537-7000; 🖥 www.arcgh.org

☎ **The Arc of King County**
206-364-6337; 🖥 www.arcofkingcounty.org

☎ **The Arc of Kitsap/Jefferson County**
360-377-3473; 🖥 www.arckj.org

☎ **The Arc of Snohomish County**
425-258-2459; 🖥 www.arcsno.org

☎ **The Arc of Spokane**
509-328-6326; 🖥 www.arc-spokane.org

☎ **The Arc of Tri-Cities**
509-946-5157; 🖥 www.arcoftricities.com

☎ **The Arc of Whatcom County** (*serving Skagit and Island Counties*)
360-715-0170; 🖥 www.arcwhatcom.org

☎ **The Arc of Yakima County**
509-453-4756 ext.228

Autism Society of Washington
The Autism Society of Washington provides information, local resources and support to families affected by autism.
☎ **1-888-ASW 4 YOU (888-279-4968)**
☎ **1-360-786-1101**
🖥 **www.autismsocietyofwa.org**

Developmental Disabilities Council (see Directory of Government Agencies—State and Local)
Disability Rights Washington (see Topical Directory—Legal)
Division of Developmental Disabilities (see Directory of Government Agencies—State and Local)

Informing Families, Building Trust
Informing Families, Building Trust (IFBT) is a partnership between the Washington State Developmental Disabilities Council, the Division of Developmental Disabilities and other key organizations. IFBT shares current news and information about the DD delivery service system.
🖥 **www.informingfamilies.org**

Disability—Mental Health

Disability Rights Washington (see Legal)

Mental Health Clubhouses
A Clubhouse is a community intentionally organized to support individuals living with the effects of mental illness. Through participation in a Clubhouse people are given the opportunities to rejoin the worlds of friendships, family, important work, employment, education, and to access the services and supports they may individually need. For the number of the Clubhouse in your area, contact your local Regional Support Network, or visit:
🖥 **www.dshs.wa.gov/Mentalhealth/clubhouses.shtml**

National Alliance on Mental Illness (NAMI)
NAMI maintains a helpline for information on mental illnesses and referrals to local groups. Local self-help groups have support and advocacy components and offer education and information about community services for families and individuals.
☎ **1-800-782-9264**
🖥 **www.nami.org**

National Suicide Prevention Lifeline is a 24-hour, toll-free suicide prevention service available to anyone in suicidal crisis. You will be routed to the closest possible crisis center in your area.
☎ **1-800-273-TALK (8255)**

Regional Support Networks (see Directory of Government Agencies—State & Local)

Disability--Physical

Disability Rights Washington (see Legal)

DIRECTORY—TOPICAL

Independent Living Centers

Independent Living Centers are part of a network of non-profit, non-residential, community-based centers, run and controlled by persons with disabilities that offer: Information and Referral; Peer counseling; Care Management; Independent living skills training; Individual and systems change advocacy; Benefits counseling; Employment readiness training; Housing referrals; and Assistive technology services.

☎ **Alliance of People with disabilities: TTY: 206-632-3456**;
Outside King Co.: **1-866-545-7055**

☎ **Alliance of People with disAbilities: East King County Office**
425-558-0993; TTY: 425-861-9588; Outside King Co.: **1-800-216-3335**

☎ **Center for Independence (CFI)**: Pierce, Thurston, S. Kitsap, Grays Harbor, Mason, and S. King Counties:
253-582-1253; TTY: 253-584-4374

☎ **Central Washington Disability Resources (CWDR)**: Kittitas, Grant, Yakima, Chelan, and Douglas Counties
509-962-9620; TTY: 1-800-240-5978

☎ **Coalition of Responsible Disabled (CORD):** Spokane, Adams, Asotin, Benton, Columbia, Ferry, Franklin, Garfield, Grant, Lincoln, Okanogan (SE), Pend Oreille, Stevens, Walla Walla, and Whitman Counties
1-877-606-2680; TTY: 509-326-6355

☎ **disability Resources of Southwest Washington (dARSW)**: Clark, Cowlitz, Skamania, and Wahkiakum Counties
360-694-6790; Fax/TTY: 800-735-2900

Tacoma Area Coalition of Individuals with Disabilities (TACID)

TACID is a non-profit organization representing people who are deaf, blind, those who have Multiple Sclerosis, and cross-disabilities groups concerned with access issues.

☎ **(253) 565-9000 ext. 12**

⌨ **www.tacid.org**

Washington State Talking Books & Braille Library

Those eligible for this service are children and adults who are residents of Washington state and who are legally blind, deaf-blind, visually impaired (cannot easily read conventional size print), have a physical disability (cannot comfortably hold books or turn pages), or have learning disability due to organic dysfunction.

☎ 1-800-542-0866

-E-

Eye Care

Seniors EyeCare Program

Formerly known as National Eye Care Project, the Seniors EyeCare Program ensures that every senior has access to medical eye care and promotes annual, dilated eye exams.

☎ 1-800-222-3937

Services for the Blind

The Washington State Department of Services for the Blind (DSB) is a state rehabilitation agency that offers assistance to persons who are blind or visually impaired.

☎ 1-800-552-7103
💻 www.dsb.wa.gov

SightLife

Operated by the Northwest Lions Foundation for Sight & Hearing, SightLife provides sight-restoring cornea implants and is one of the leading eye banks in the nation.

☎ 1-800-847-5786
💻 www.sightlife.org

-G-

Government Agencies (see Directory of Government Agencies—Federal, State and Local)

-H-

Health Care

Medicaid (see Directory of Government Agencies—State and Local)

Medicare (see Directory of Government Agencies—Federal)

Statewide Health Insurance Advisors--SHIBA (see Directory of Government Agencies—State and Local)

Transportation for Persons Receiving Medicaid (see Transportation)

TRICARE
TRICARE is a health care program for active-duty service members, retirees, and their families. The uniformed services determine who is eligible for TRICARE coverage.
☎ 1-866-773-0404
🖳 www.tricare4u.com

Housing

Home Energy & Weatherization Assistance
A statewide network of 27 local community-based nonprofit organizations, known as Community Action Programs (or Councils) provide energy and weatherization services through a grant program.
☎ 360-725-2905
🖳 www.liheapwa.org

Public Housing Agency
Public Housing Agencies administer affordable housing programs for low-income people—including seniors and persons with disabilities. To find the housing agency nearest you, call the US Department of Housing and Urban Development Information and Resource Center.
☎ 1-800-955-2232

Washington Information Network (WIN 2-1-1)
A directory of health and human service program resources for food banks, emergency shelters, transportation, rent, in-home care services and more.
☎ 211
🖳 www.liheapwa.org

-I-

In-Home Support

Home Care Association of Washington online directory helps consumers find and choose providers of home care and hospice services. The database consists of home care and hospice agencies that are HCAW members.
- ☎ 1-425-775-8120
- 💻 www.hcaw.org

Home Care Referral Registry

If you receive Medicaid Personal Care, contact the Home Care Referral Registry in your area. The Home Care Referral Registry can match your in-home care needs with pre-qualified, pre-screened individual providers who are ready to work.
- ☎ 1-800-970-5456
- 💻 www.hcrr.wa.gov

National Association of Home Care Agencies

The National Association of Home Care Agencies provides a database of home care and hospice agencies.
- ☎ 202-547-7424
- 💻 www.nahc.org

Washington State Home Care Coalition

The Washington State Home Care Coalition is a membership association which was formed in 1979 as the "Chore Coalition" to provide guidance and advocacy for home care agencies statewide.
- ☎ 360-896-9695
- ☎ 503-221-7441
- 💻 www.cdmservices.net

Washington State Hospice and Palliative Care Organization (WSHPCO)

WSHPCO is a non-profit organization of hospice and palliative care providers. For a listing of providers, visit the website and click on the Find a Provider button.
- ☎ 1-866-661-3739
- ☎ 253-661-3739
- 💻 www.wshpco.org

DIRECTORY—TOPICAL

-L-

Legal

Coordinated Legal Education, Advice and Referral System (CLEAR, CLEAR*Sr)
CLEAR provides free legal assistance to low-income people with civil legal problems (Note: assistance is provided to seniors age 60 and older regardless of income or resources). Interpreter services are available.
☎ Inside King County: 206-464-1519; Outside King County: 1-888-201-1014

CLEAR*Sr (for people over 60)
☎ 1-888-387-7111; 1-888-201-9737 (TTY)
🖥 www.nwjustice.org

Disability Rights Washington
Disability Rights Washington is a nonprofit organization providing legal advocacy services to Washington residents with disabilities. Services include: Information and referral; Legal representation; Abuse or neglect investigation. Serves all people with disabilities.
☎ 1-800-562-2702
☎ 1-800-905-0209
Interpreters available in over 200 languages via AT&T Language Line.
🖥 www.disabilityrightswa.org

Dispute Resolution Centers Elder Mediation Program
The Elder Mediation Program within Dispute Resolution Centers assists elders, their families and caregivers with resolving conflict that may arise around issues of autonomy, housing, health care or end-of-life decisions. Trained mediators will meet with families throughout the region. Sliding fee. No one is turned away due to lack of funds.
🖥 www.resolutionwa.org

Living Will Registry
The Washington State Department of Health offers a free online registry that lets Washington State residents have their end-of-life preferences available online to authorized health care providers.
🖥 www.doh.wa.gov/livingwill

DIRECTORY--TOPICAL

National Academy of Elder Law Attorneys (NAELA)
Provides an online directory of its members to locate attorneys that deal with legal issues affecting elderly and disabled adults.
⌨ **www.naela.com**

Washington LawHelp
Washington LawHelp is an online self-help resource for a variety of legal issues such as elder law, housing, immigration, health and government benefits, etc.
⌨ **www.washingtonlawhelp.org**

Washington Bar Association
For information about wills, visit:
⌨ **www.wsba.org**

-M-

Meals & Food Assistance

Home Delivered Meals are offered to seniors and persons with disabilities who are unable to leave their homes.
☎ Contact your local Area Agency on Aging to find the organization or agency contracted to provide meal delivery services.

Group Meals. Also known as congregate meals, group meals are offered at various community locations, such as a senior center, tribal center or community center.
☎ Contact your local Area Agency on Aging for a list of on-site meal programs near you. (See Government—State & Local)

Washington Basic Food Program
Once known as "food stamps," the Washington Basic Food Program issues Benefits Transfer Cards, also called "Quest Cards." Contact the Aging and Disability Services Administration Helpline for the Community Services Office (CSO) nearest you:
☎ **1-877-501-2233**
Or apply Online:
⌨ **www.DSHS.wa.gov,** go to: "help with food".

DIRECTORY—TOPICAL

Food Banks

Hundreds of food banks exist throughout the state. No one is turned away.
To find a food bank near you, contact Northwest Harvest:

☎ **1-800-722-6924**

🖥 **www.northwestharvest.org**

🖥 **www.resourcehouse.info/Win211**

For a statewide map of food banks, visit:

🖥 **www.cted.wa.gov/maps**

Senior Farmer's Market Nutrition Coordinators

The Senior Farmer's Market Nutrition Program is administered by DSHS Aging and Disability Services Administration in partnership with the Washington State Department of Health, Area Agencies on Aging, Washington State Farmers Market Association, Washington Association of Senior Nutrition Programs, Department of Agriculture.

☎ **Adams, Chelan, Douglas, Grant, Lincoln, Okanogan**
509-886-0700 or 1-800-572-4459

☎ **Asotin, Benton, Columbia, Franklin, Garfield, Kittitas, Yakima, Walla Walla**
509-965-0105 or 1-877-965-2582

☎ **Clallam, Jefferson, Grays Harbor, Pacific**
360-379-5064 or 1-866-720-4863

☎ **Clark, Cowlitz, Klickitat, Skamania, Wahkiakum**
360-694-8144 or 1-888-637-6060

☎ **Colville Confederated Tribes**
509-634-2759

☎ **King**
206-448-3110 or 1-888-435-3377

☎ **Kitsap**
360-337-7068 or 1-800-562-6418

☎ **Lewis, Mason, Thurston**
360-664-3162 ext. 146 or 1-888-545-0910

☎ **Pierce**
253-798-7376 or 1-800-642-5769

☎ **Snohomish**
425-388-7218

☎ **Spokane, Whitman, Ferry, Pend Oreille, Stevens**

509-458-2509

☎ **Whatcom, Skagit, San Juan, Island**
360-676-6749 or 1-800-585-6749

☎ **Yakima Indian Nation:**
509-865-7164

-N-

Nursing Homes

(See Residential Care)

-P-

Prescription Drugs

Consumer Reports Best Buy Drugs

Best Buy Drugs is a public education project that offers free guidance for consumers on prescription medicines. It will help you talk to your doctor about prescription drugs, and find the most effective and safe drugs that also give you the best value for your health care dollar.

💻   **www.consumerreports.org/health/best-buy-drugs/index.htm**

Washington Prescription Drug Program

WPDP is a new prescription drug discount program open to all Washington State residents who do not have prescription drug insurance coverage, or whose insurance does not cover all their prescription drug needs.

☎   **206-521-2027 or 1-800-442-2183**
💻   **www.rx.wa.gov**

Statewide Health Insurance Benefits Advisors—SHIBA (see Directory of Government Agencies—State & Local)

-R-

Residential Care

Residential Care facilities (Adult Family Homes, Boarding Homes, Nursing Homes) provide varying levels of care for seniors and individuals with disabilities. For a list of facilities near you, contact Home and Community Services (see Government—State & Local) if you receive Medicaid.

Senior Housing Locator (powered by SNAP for Seniors)
Find adult family homes, assisted living, nursing & rehabilitation homes, Continuing Care Retirement Communities (CCRC's) and independent living retirement communities.
🖥 **www.seniorhousinglocator.org**

Compare Nursing Homes in Washington State

Concerned about a nursing home's performance? The U.S. Dept of Health and Human Services offers great online information about the past performance of every Medicare and Medicaid certified nursing home in the country. Visit: www.medicare.gov and click on "Compare Home Health Agencies in Your Area."

-S-

Safety

Personal Emergency Response Systems
Home medical alert systems, sometimes called Personal Emergency Response Systems are very helpful for adults who have frequent falls and/or fear of falls; limited mobility; medication concerns; or medical conditions. Below are examples of businesses that sell medical alert systems. Installation and monitoring fees may apply (unless you are receiving the service through a publicly funded source such as COPES).

☎ ADT Companion Service: **1-800-209-7599;** 🖥 **www.adt.com**

☎ Lifeline: **1-800-380-3111;** 🖥 **www.lifelinesys.com**

☎ Link-to-Life: **1-888-337-5433;** 💻 **www.link-to-life.com**

Seniors

American Association of Retired Persons (AARP)

AARP is a nonprofit membership organization of persons 50 and older dedicated to addressing their needs and interests. Learn more about this organization.

☎ **1-888-OUR-AARP (1-888-687-2277)**

💻 **www.aarp.org**

Area Agency on Aging (see Directory of Government Agencies—State & Local)

Eldercare Locator

Eldercare Locator is a free service of the Administration on Aging. Call from anywhere in the county to connect with state and local agencies, or go online and search from your computer.

☎ **1-800-677-1116**

💻 **www.eldercare.gov**

National Council on Aging

The National Council on Aging (NCOA) is a nonprofit organization that helps older people remain healthy and independent, find jobs, increase access to benefits programs, and discover meaningful ways to continue contributing to society. NCOA provides BenefitsCheckUp, a free online tool for figuring out what benefits you may qualify to receive.

💻 **www.ncoa.org**

Senior Information & Assistance (see Directory of Government Agencies—State & Local)

DIRECTORY—TOPICAL

-T-

Transportation

Medical Transportation

For individuals who are eligible to receive Medicaid services, The Washington State Department of Social and Health Services will pay for non-emergency medical transportation. To find the Medicaid-contracted transportation provider in your area, call the Medical Assistance Helpline:

☎ **1-800-562-3022**

☎ **1-800-848-5429 (TTY/TDD)**

-V-

Veterans

Paralyzed Veterans of America

Aggressive advocates for an accessible America.

☎ **1-800-336-9782**

Northwest Chapter for Paralyzed Veterans of America

☎ **206-241-1843**

💻 **www.nwpva.org**

National Association of County Veteran Service Officers (NACVSO)

NACVSO provides assistance in obtaining veterans' benefits and answers questions regarding rules and regulations concerning veterans. For veterans and family members.

💻 **www.nacvso.org**

U.S. Department of Veterans Affairs (see Directory of Government Agencies—Federal)

Washington State Department of Veterans Affairs (see Directory of Government Agencies—State & Local)

Wills and Trusts

(See Topical Directory—Legal)

DIRECTORY--TOPICAL

Directory of Government Agencies

Federal Government

Administration on Aging

The Administration on Aging is the Federal focal point and advocate agency for older persons and their concerns. AoA sponsors the ElderCare Locator, a free service that connects you with eldercare services in your community.

☎ **1-800-677-1116**

💻 **www.aoa.gov**

Medicare

Medicare provides health insurance for people age 65 or older, under age 65 with certain disabilities, and any age with End-Stage Renal Disease.

☎ **1-800-633-4227 or 1-877-486-2048 (TTY)**

💻 **www.medicare.gov**

Social Security Administration

Contact Social Security to apply for retirement or disability benefits. For the number of the SSA field office nearest you, call SSA toll-free and request the number through the automated system. Social Security has a toll-free number that operates from 7 a.m. to 7 p.m., Monday through Friday:

☎ **1-800-772-1213 or 1-800-325-0778 (TTY)**

💻 **www.ssa.gov**

Veterans Administration

If you are a veteran or have served in the U.S. military, call the U.S. Department of Veterans Affairs (VA) for information about veterans' benefits and services available in your area.

☎ **1-800-827-1000**

💻 **www.va.gov**

State and Local Government

-A-

Adult Protective Services

Adult Protective Services (APS) investigates complaints of abuse against vulnerable adults living in their own home or somewhere other than a residential care facility. Calls can be made anonymously.

☎ **Region 1:** Spokane, Grant, Okanogan, Adams, Chelan, Douglas, Lincoln, Ferry, Stevens, Whitman and Pend Oreille
1-800-459-0421; TTY: 1-509-568-3086

☎ **Region 2:** Yakima, Kittitas, Benton, Franklin, Walla Walla, Columbia, Garfield and Asotin
1-877-389-3013; TTY: 1-800-973-5456

☎ **Region 3:** Snohomish, Skagit, Island, San Juan, Whatcom
1-800-487-0416; TTY: 1-800-843-8058

☎ **Region 4:** King
1-866-221-4909; TTY: 1-800-977-5456

☎ **Region 5:**
Pierce
1-800-442-5129; TTY: 1-800-688-1165
Kitsap
1-888-833-4925; TTY: 1-800-688-1169

☎ **Region 6:** Thurston, Lewis, Clallam, Jefferson, Grays Harbor, Pacific, Wahkiakum, Cowlitz, Skamania, Klickitat, Clark
1-877-734-6277; TTY: 1-800-672-7091

Aging & Disability Services Administration

Call the Aging & Disability Services Administration Helpline to ask for information about your local: Area Agency on Aging; Division of Developmental Disabilities; Home and Community Office; Licensed Adult Family Homes, Boarding Home and Nursing Home.
☎ **1-800-422-3263**
⌨ **www.adsa.dshs.wa.gov**

Area Agency on Aging
Senior Information & Assistance, Family Caregiver Support Program, Case management services for seniors and adults with disabilities. (Note: Some AAA's have a different number for Senior Information and Assistance.)

☎ **Adams County: 509-886-0700 or 1-800-572-4459**
  Senior I&A: **509-766-2568 or 877-380-5787**

☎ **Asotin County: 509-965-0105 or 1-877-965-2582;**
  Senior I&A: **509-758-2355**

☎ **Benton County: 509-965-0105 or 1-877-965-2582;**
  Senior I&A: **509-735-0315**

☎ **Chelan County: 509-886-0700 or 1-800-572-4459**

☎ **Clallam County: 1-866-720-4863;**
  Senior I&A:
  360-452-3221 or 1-800-801-0070 (Sequim)
  360-374-9496 or 1-888-571-6559 (Forks)

☎ **Clark County: 360-735-5720 or 1-888-637-6060;**
  Senior I&A: **360-694-8144**

☎ **Columbia County: 509-965-0105 or 1-877-965-2582;**
  Senior I&A: **509-382-4787**

☎ **Colville Confederated Tribes: 509-634-2758 or 1-888-881-7684;**

☎ **Cowlitz County: 360-694-8144 or 1-888-637-6060;**
  Senior I&A: **360-577-4929 or 1-800-682-2406**

☎ **Douglas County: 509-886-0700 or 1-800-572-4459**

☎ **Ferry County: 509-458-2509;**
  Senior I&A: **509-775-3341**

☎ **Franklin County: 509-965-0105 or 1-877-965-2582;**
  Senior I&A: **509-545-3459**

☎ **Garfield County: 509-965-0105 or 1-877-965-2582;**
  Senior I&A: **509-843-3563**

☎ **Grant County: 509-886-0700 or 1-800-572-4459**
  Senior I&A: **509-766-2568, 1-877-380-5787**

☎ **Grays Harbor County: 1-866-720-4863;**
  Senior I&A: **360-532-0520 or 1-800-801-0060**

DIRECTORY—GOVERNMENT STATE & LOCAL

☎ **Island County: 360-676-6749 or 1-800-585-6749;**
Senior I&A:
360-675-0311 (Oak Harbor)
360-678-4886 (Coupeville)
360-321-1600 (South Whidbey)
360-387-6201 (Camano Island)

☎ **Jefferson County: 1-866-720-4863;**
Senior I&A: **360-385-2552 or 1-800-801-0050**

☎ **King County: 206-684-0660 or 1-888-435-3377;**
Senior I&A: **206-448-3110 or 1-888-435-3377**

☎ **Kitsap County: 360-337-5700 or 1-800-562-6418**

☎ **Kittitas County: 509-965-0105 or 1-877-965-2582;**
Senior I&A: **509-925-8765 or 1-877-401-2583**

☎ **Klickitat County: 360-694-8144 or 1-888-637-6060;**
Senior I&A: **1-800-447-7858, or**
509-493-3068 (White Salmon)
509-773-3757 (Goldendale)

☎ **Lewis County: 360-664-2168 or 1-888-545-0910;**
Senior I&A:
360-748-2288 or 1-888-702-4464 (Chehalis)
360-496-6300 or 1-800-247-5872 (Morton)

☎ **Lincoln County: 509-886-0700 or 1-800-572-4459**
Senior I&A: **509-766-2568, 1-877-380-5787**

☎ **Mason County: 360-664-2168 or 1-888-545-0910;**
Senior I&A: **360-427-2225 or 1-877-227-4696**

☎ **Okanogan County:**
509-886-0700 or 1-800-572-4459;
Senior I&A: **509-826-7452 or 1-888-437-4147**

☎ **Pacific County: 360-379-5064 or 1-866-720-4863**
Senior I&A:
360-942-2177 or 1-888-571-6557 (Raymond)
360-642-3634 or 1-888-571-6558 (Long Beach)

☎ **Pend Oreille County: 509-458-2509;**
Senior I&A: **509-684-8421**

DIRECTORY—GOVERNMENT STATE & LOCAL

☎ **Pierce County: 253-798-7236 or 1-800-642-5769;**
Aging & Disability Resource Center: **253-798-4600 or 1-800-562-0332**

☎ **San Juan County: 360-676-6749 or 1-800-585-6749;**
Senior I&A:
360-376-2677 (Orcas, Blakely, Waldron)
360-378-2677 (San Juan, Brown, Henry, Stuart)
360-468-2421 (Lopez, Shaw, Center, Decatur)

☎ **Skagit County: 360-676-6749 or 1-800-585-6749;**
Senior I&A: **360-428-1301**

☎ **Skamania County: 360-694-8144 or 1-888-637-6060;**
Senior I&A: **509-427-3990**

☎ **Snohomish County:**
425-513-1900 or 1-800-422-2024 or 425-347-7997 (TDD)

☎ **Spokane County: 509-458-2509;**
Senior I&A: **509-458-7450**

☎ **Stevens County: 509-458-2509;**
Senior I&A: **509-684-8421 or 1-800-873-5889**

☎ **Thurston County: 360-664-2168 or 1-888-545-0910**

☎ **Wahkiakum County: 360-694-8144 or 1-888-637-6060;**
Senior I&A: **360-577-4929 or 1-800-682-2406**

☎ **Walla Walla: 509-965-0105 or 1-877-965-2582**;
Senior I&A: **509-529-6470 or 1-888-769-2582**

☎ **Whatcom County: 360-676-6749 or 1-800-585-6749;**
Senior I&A: **360-738-2500**

☎ **Whitman County: 509-458-2509**;
Senior I&A: **509-397-4305 or 1-800809-3351**

☎ **Yakima County: 509-965-0105 or 1-877-965-2582**;
Senior I&A:
509-469-0500 or 1-866-891-2582 (Yakima County)
509-829-3905 or 1-888-549-2582 (Lower Yakima Valley)

☎ **Yakima Nation: 509-865-7164**
509-865-5121 ext. 481

DIRECTORY—GOVERNMENT STATE & LOCAL

-B-

Services for the Blind

The Washington State Department of Services for the Blind (DSB) is a state rehabilitation agency that offers assistance to persons who are blind or visually impaired.

☎ **1-800-552-7103**

☎ **TTY 1-206-721-4056**

💻 **www.dsb.wa.gov**

-C-

Community Services Office

Local Community Services Offices (CSO) provide many DSHS services, such as Medical Assistance (Medicaid) and food assistance (Quest Card). For the number of the CSO office nearest you, look in the Blue Pages of your phone book, under State Government/Social and Health Services/Community Services Office. Or, visit the Department of Social and Health Services website and click on the link to available services.

💻 **www.dshs.wa.gov**.

Complaint Resolution Unit

Contact the Complaint Resolution Unit if the person that you suspect is being abused or neglected is living in a nursing home, boarding home, or adult family home.

☎ **1-800-562-6078**

-D-

Deaf and Hard of Hearing, Office of

The Office of the Deaf and Hard of Hearing (ODHH) provides services to the deaf, hard of hearing and deaf-blind communities throughout Washington State. ODHH contracts with five regional service centers with seven offices, located in Seattle, Tacoma, Vancouver, Pasco, Spokane, and Bellingham, to provide case management, advocacy, workshops, information and referral, education and training, and outreach services to clients and their families.

☎ **360-902-8000 Voice/TTY or 1-800-422-7930 Voice/TTY**

Developmental Disabilities Council

The Washington State Developmental Disabilities Council is appointed by the Governor to promote a comprehensive system of services, and serve as an advocate and a planning body for Washington State's citizens with developmental disabilities. The DDC funds projects, such as Informing Families, Building Trusts, which provide information related to developmental disability policies and services.

☎ **1-800-634-4473**

💻 **www.ddc.wa.gov**

Division of Developmental Disabilities

The Division of Developmental Disabilities, is a division within Aging and Disability Services, provides services and supports to eligible children and adults with developmental disabilities.

☎ **Region 1:** Adams, Chelan, Douglas, Ferry, Grant, Lincoln, Okanogan, Pend Oreille, Spokane, Stevens, Whitman.
509-329-2900; TTY: 509-568-3038; 1-800-462-0624

☎ **Region 2:** Asotin, Benton, Columbia, Franklin, Garfield, Kittitas, Klickitat, Walla Walla, Yakima
509-225-4620; TTY: 509-454-4321; 1-800-822-7840

☎ **Region 3:** Island, San Juan, Skagit, Snohomish, Whatcom
425-339-4833; TTY: 425-339-4850; 1-800-788-2053

☎ **Region 4:** King
206-568-5700; TTY: 206-720-3325; 1-800-314-3296

☎ **Region 5:** Kitsap, Pierce
253-404-6500; TTY: 253-572-7381; 1-800-248-0949

☎ **Region 6:** Clallam, Clark, Cowlitz, Grays Harbor, Jefferson, Lewis, Mason, Pacific, Skamania, Thurston, Wahkiakum
360-725-4250; TTY: 360-586-4719; 1-800-339-8227

Division of Vocational Rehabilitation

The Division of Vocational Rehabilitation is a statewide resource that helps people with disabilities obtain and retain employment. It provides information and referral services for independent living and individual counseling. To be connected to your local DVR office, call:

☎ **1-800-637-5627**

💻 **www1.dshs.wa.gov/dvr/**

DIRECTORY—GOVERNMENT STATE & LOCAL

-H-

Home Care Referral Registry

The Home Care Referral Registry is used to match needs of Washington State residents who receive publicly funded long term in-home care with pre-screened and pre-qualified in-home care workers.

☎ **1-800-970-5456**

💻 **www.hcrr.wa.gov**

Home and Community Services

Home and Community Services is a division within Aging & Disability Services Administration that helps adults who may need help paying for long term care due to a medical conditions or disability. Also provides assistance in applying for Medicaid.

☎ **Region 1:** Spokane, Grant, Okanogan, Adams, Chelan, Douglas, Lincoln, Ferry, Stevens, Whitman, Pend Oreille Counties
1-800-459-0421

☎ **Region 2:** Yakima, Kittitas, Benton, Franklin, Walla Walla, Columbia, Garfield, and Asotin Counties
1-800-822-2097

☎ **Region 3:** Snohomish, Skagit, Island, San Juan, and Whatcom Counties
1-800-487-0416

☎ **Region 4:** King County
1-800-346-9257

☎ **Region 5:**
1-800-442-5129 (Pierce County)
1-800-422-7114 (Kitsap County)

☎ **Region 6:** Thurston, Mason, Lewis, Clallam, Jefferson, Grays Harbor, Pacific, Wahkiakum, Cowlitz, Skamania, Klickitat, and Clark Counties
1-800-462-4957

-L-

Long Term Care Ombudsman

A Long-Term Care Ombudsman responds to complaints about Adult Family Home, Boarding Homes and Nursing Homes.

☎ **1-800-562-6028**

-M-

Medical Assistance/Medicaid
Medicaid is a state and federal government health insurance program available to people with very limited income and resources. Apply online or contact your Community Services Office to apply in person.
Medical Assistance Helpline (for current Medicaid recipients):
☎ **1-800-562-3022; TTY/TDD: 1-800-848-5429**
💻 **www.adsa.dshs.wa.gov/pubinfo/benefits/medicaid.htm**

Mental Health Division – Regional Support Networks
Within the Washington State mental health system, county government agencies and 145 private and non-profit organizations provide treatment for most of Washington's estimated 188,100 adults and 74,000 children with mental illnesses. Counties, and their non-government providers, are organized into 13 Regional Support Networks:

☎ **Chelan-Douglas RSN**
   509-886-6318 or 1-877-563-3678
   24-Hour Crisis Line: 509-662-7105

☎ **Clark County RSN**
   360-397-2130 or 1-866-666-5070
   24-Hour Crisis Line: 1-800-626-8137

☎ **Greater Columbia Behavioral Health RSN:** Serving Asotin, Benton, Columbia, Franklin, Garfield, Kittitas, Klickitat, Skamania, Walla Walla, Whitman and Yakima Counties.
   509-735-8681; 1-800-795-9296
   24-Hour Crisis Lines:
   Asotin: 1-888-475-5665
   Benton-Franklin: 1-800-783-0544
   Columbia: 1-866-382-1164
   Garfield: 1-888-475-5665
   Kittitas: 509-925-9861 or 1-800-572-8122
   Klickitat: 509-733-5801 or 1-800-572-8122
   Skamania: 509-427-3850
   Walla Walla: 509-522-3278
   Whitman: 1-866-871-6385
   Yakima: 509-575-4200 or 1-800-572-8122
   Yakima Children: 509-576-0934 or 1-800-500-0934

☎ **Grays Harbor County RSN**
360-532-8665; 1-800-464-7277
24-Hour Crisis Line: 1-800-685-6556

☎ **King County RSN**
206-296-5213; 1-800-790-8049
24-Hour Crisis Line: 1-866-427-4747

☎ **North Central WA RSN:** Serving Adams, Grant, Okanogan, Ferry, Lincoln, Pend Oreille and Stevens Counties
509-754-6577; 1-800-251-5350
24-Hour Crisis Lines:
Adams County(collect): 509-488-5611
Ferry County: 1-866-268-5105
Grant County: 1-877-467-4303
Okanogan County: 1-866-826-6191
Pend Oreille: 1-866-847-8540
Stevens & Lincoln Counties: 1-888-380-6823

☎ **North Sound Mental Health Administration RSN:** Serving Island, San Juan, Skagit, Snohomish and Whatcom Counties
1-800-684-3555
24-Hour Crisis Line: 1-800-584-3578

☎ **Peninsula RSN - Serving Clallam, Jefferson and Kitsap Counties**
360-337-4886; 1-800-525-5637;
24-Hour Crisis Lines:
Kitsap County: 360-479-3033 or 1-800-843-4793
East Jefferson County: 360-385-0321 or 1-800-659-0321
East Clallam County: 360-452-4500
West Jefferson County: 360-374-5011
West Clallam County: 360-374-5011;(Non-Business hours): 360-374-6271

☎ **Pierce County**
253-798-7202;1-800-531-0508
24-Hour Crisis Line: 1-800-576-7764

☎ **Southwest RSN:** Serving Cowlitz County
360-501-1201; 1-800-347-6092
24-Hour Crisis Line: 1-800-803-8833

☎ **Spokane County RSN**
509-477-5722; 1-800-273-5864
24-Hour Crisis Line: 1-877-678-4428

DIRECTORY—GOVERNMENT STATE & LOCAL

☎ **Thurston-Mason RSN -**
360-786-5830; 1-800-658-4105; TDD: 360-786-5602 or 1-800-658-6384

24-Hour Crisis Line: 1-800-754-1338

☎ **Timberlands RSN:** Serving Lewis, Pacific and Wahkiakum Counties
360-795-3118; 1-800-392-6298
24-Hour Crisis Lines:
Lewis County: 1-800-559-6696
Pacific County: 1-800-884-2298
Wahkiakum County: 1-800-635-5989

-S-

Statewide Health Insurance Advisors (SHIBA)
The Statewide Health Insurance Benefits Advisors (SHIBA) HelpLine provides for all Washington residents, **free** health insurance education, assistance, and advocacy. SHIBA HelpLine assists consumers with choices and problems involving private health insurance as well as many government programs.
☎ 1-800-562-6900; TDD: 360-586-0241
💻 www.insurance.wa.gov/shiba

-V-

Washington State Department of Veterans Affairs
☎ 1-800-562-0132; 360-725-2199 (TDD)
💻 www.dva.wa.gov

DIRECTORY—GOVERNMENT STATE & LOCAL

The **Home Care Referral Registry of Washington State** matches those who need in-home long-term care services with pre-qualified, pre-screened individual providers that are ready to work.

For more information about the Home Care Referral Registry call 800-970-5456.

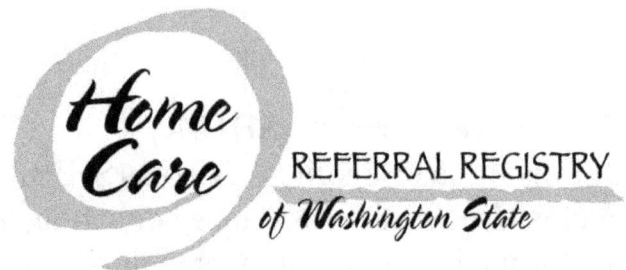

www.ingramcontent.com/pod-product-compliance
Lightning Source LLC
Chambersburg PA
CBHW081134170526
45165CB00008B/2666